Lecture Notes in Computer Science 7096

Commenced Publication in 1973
Founding and Former Series Editors:
Gerhard Goos, Juris Hartmanis, and Jan van Leeuwen

Editorial Board

David Hutchison
Lancaster University, UK

Takeo Kanade
Carnegie Mellon University, Pittsburgh, PA, USA

Josef Kittler
University of Surrey, Guildford, UK

Jon M. Kleinberg
Cornell University, Ithaca, NY, USA

Alfred Kobsa
University of California, Irvine, CA, USA

Friedemann Mattern
ETH Zurich, Switzerland

John C. Mitchell
Stanford University, CA, USA

Moni Naor
Weizmann Institute of Science, Rehovot, Israel

Oscar Nierstrasz
University of Bern, Switzerland

C. Pandu Rangan
Indian Institute of Technology, Madras, India

Bernhard Steffen
TU Dortmund University, Germany

Madhu Sudan
Microsoft Research, Cambridge, MA, USA

Demetri Terzopoulos
University of California, Los Angeles, CA, USA

Doug Tygar
University of California, Berkeley, CA, USA

Gerhard Weikum
Max Planck Institute for Informatics, Saarbruecken, Germany

Mika Rautiainen Timo Korhonen
Edward Mutafungwa Eila Ovaska
Artem Katasonov Antti Evesti
Heikki Ailisto Aaron Quigley
Jonna Häkkilä Natasa Milic-Frayling
Jukka Riekki (Eds.)

Grid and Pervasive Computing Workshops

International Workshops, S3E, HWTS, Doctoral Colloquium
Held in Conjunction with GPC 2011
Oulu, Finland, May 11-13, 2011
Revised Selected Papers

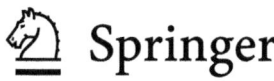 Springer

Volume Editors

Mika Rautiainen
Jukka Riekki
University of Oulu, Finland
{mika.rautiainen; jukka.riekki}@ee.oulu.fi

Timo Korhonen
Edward Mutafungwa
Aalto University, Helsinki, Finland
timo.korhonen@aalto.fi; edward.mutafungwa@tkk.fi

Eila Ovaska
Artem Katasonov
Antti Evesti
Heikki Ailisto
VTT Technical Research Centre of Finland, Oulu, Finland
{eila.ovaska; artem.katasonov; antti.evesti; heikki.ailisto}@vtt.fi

Aaron Quigley
University of St. Andrews, UK; aquigley@st-andrews.ac.uk

Jonna Häkkilä
Nokia Research Center, Oulu, Finland; jonna.hakkila@nokia.com

Natasa Milic-Frayling
Microsoft Research, Cambridge, UK; natasamf@microsoft.com

ISSN 0302-9743　　　　　　　　　　e-ISSN 1611-3349
ISBN 978-3-642-27915-7　　　　　　e-ISBN 978-3-642-27916-4
DOI 10.1007/978-3-642-27916-4
Springer Heidelberg Dordrecht London New York

Library of Congress Control Number: 2011945034

CR Subject Classification (1998): C.2, H.4, H.3, H.5, D.2, I.2

LNCS Sublibrary: SL 3 – Information Systems and Application, incl. Internet/Web
and HCI

Typesetting: Camera-ready by author, data conversion by Scientific Publishing Services, Chennai, India

Printed on acid-free paper

Springer is part of Springer Science+Business Media (www.springer.com)

Preface

GPC 2011 was the sixth in a conference series that provides a forum for researchers and practitioners in all areas of grid and cloud computing as well as pervasive computing. Two workshops were held in conjunction with the GPC 2011 conference: the International Workshop on Health and Well-being Technologies and Services for Elderly (HWTS 2011) and the International Workshop on Self-Managing Solutions for Smart Environments (S3E 2011). In addition, PhD students received valuable feedback for their doctoral studies in the doctoral colloquium from the colloquium panelists and their peers.

The conference would not have been possible without the support of many people and organizations that helped in various ways to make it a success. In particular, we would like to thank Infotech Oulu and the MOTIVE program of the Academy of Finland for their financial support. We are also grateful to the workshop organizers, committee members and the external reviewers for their dedication in reviewing the submissions. We also thank the authors for their efforts in writing and revising their papers, and we thank Springer for publishing the proceedings.

October 2011

Mika Rautiainen
Timo Korhonen
Edward Mutafungwa
Eila Ovaska
Artem Katasonov
Antti Evesti
Heikki Ailisto
Aaron Quigley
Jonna Häkkilä
Natasa Milic-Frayling
Jukka Riekki

Organization
GPC 2011

Steering Committee

Hai Jin (Chair)	Huazhong University of Science and Technology, China
Nabil Abdennadher	University of Applied Sciences, Switzerland
Christophe Cerin	University of Paris XIII, France
Sajal K. Das	The University of Texas at Arlington, USA
Jean-Luc Gaudiot	University of California - Irvine, USA
Kuan-Ching Li	Providence University, Taiwan
Cho-Li Wang	The University of Hong Kong, China
Chao-Tung Yang	Tunghai University, Taiwan

Conference Chairs

Jukka Riekki	University of Oulu, Finland
Depei Qian	Beihang University, China
Mika Ylianttila	University of Oulu, Finland

Program Chairs

Jukka Riekki	University of Oulu, Finland
Timo Korhonen	Aalto University, Finland
Minyi Guo	Shanghai Jiaotong University, China

Workshop and Tutorial Chairs

Jiehan Zhou	University of Oulu, Finland
Mika Rautiainen	University of Oulu, Finland
Zhonghong Ou	Aalto University, Finland

Workshop on Self-Managing Solutions for Smart Environments (S3E 2011)
Preface

This volume contains papers presented at S3E 2011: the First International Workshop on Self-Managing Solutions for Smart Environments, held on May 11, 2011, as part of the 6th International Conference on Grid and Pervasive Computing (GPC) at the University of Oulu, Finland.

Smart environments are small worlds where different kinds of smart devices are continuously working to make inhabitants' lives more comfortable, safe, or economic. Smart homes, smart workspaces, smart cars aim at automating repetitive tasks and increasing their efficiency, at raising humans' awareness of the state of the environment, and at allowing more control over this state. Smart environments as a research area is at the intersection of such fields as ubiquitous computing and the Web of Things, intelligent systems, and semantic interoperability. The S3E workshop focused on how to manage the inherent dynamism of smart environments and to provide enhanced intelligence for their proactive behavior.

The workshop received nine submissions originating from six countries. Each submission was reviewed by at least three Program Committee members, and five papers were selected. The problems, which the papers presented at the workshop focused on, included context-awareness, activity recognition, machine learning, security and cross-device interoperability in smart environments.

In addition to the presentation of the regular papers, the workshop also included a keynote speech by Vagan Terziyan, Professor in Distributed Systems at the University of Jyväskylä, Finland. The abstract of this keynote is also contained in this volume. In addition, the workshop included a demo session.

We would like to thank the members of the Program Committee for helping in assuring the quality of the workshop program. The organization of the workshop was in part supported by the project SOFIA, which is a part of EU's ARTEMIS Joint Undertaking.

May 2011

Eila Ovaska
Artem Katasonov
Antti Evesti

Organization

Workshop Chairs

Eila Ovaska — VTT Technical Research Centre of Finland, Finland

Artem Katasonov — VTT Technical Research Centre of Finland, Finland

Antti Evesti — VTT Technical Research Centre of Finland, Finland

Program Committee

Muhammad Ali Babar — IT University of Copenhagen, Denmark

Paolo Bellavista — University of Bologna, Italy

Jukka Honkola — Innorange Oy, Finland

Kai Koskimies — Tampere University of Technology, Finland

Ville Könönen — VTT Technical Research Centre of Finland, Finland

Tomi Männistö — Helsinki University of Technology, Finland

Tanir Ozcelebi — Eindhoven University of Technology, The Netherlands

Leonardo Querzoni — Sapienza University of Rome, Italy

Claudia Raibulet — University of Milan-Bicocca, Italy

Reijo Savola — VTT Technical Research Centre of Finland, Finland

Aly Syed — NXP Semiconductors, The Netherlands

Additional Reviewers

Sachin Bhardwaj — Eindhoven University of Technology, The Netherlands

Aravind Kota Gopalakrishna — Eindhoven University of Technology, The Netherlands

Sunder Rao — Eindhoven University of Technology, The Netherlands

Workshop on Health and Well-Being Technologies and Services for Elderly (HWTS 2011)
Preface

The International Workshop on Health and Well-Being Technologies and Services for Elderly (HWTS 2011) was held in conjunction with the 6th International Conference on Grid and Pervasive Computing (GPC 2011) in Oulu, Finland, during May 11–13, 2011. This volume contains the full papers that were presented at the Workshop.

We received ten submissions that were each reviewed by two or three Technical Program Committee (TPC) members. Finally, the TPC selected seven full regular papers for presentation at the conference and inclusion in this LNCS volume. The papers selected for presentation highlighted some novel approaches and/or innovative implementations that are highly relevant from the perspective of e-Health services and technologies, particularly those targeting the fast-rising elderly population. To that end, the papers in this volume are grouped into two categories: those that address User Interface and Service Designs for Elderly Users, and those that describe the implementations of Telehealth Systems.

In addition to the regular paper presentations, three high-quality keynotes were also presented during HWTS 2011. The keynotes included: a presentation of the state-of-the-art research, development and innovation activities carried out by the TRIL centre (Technology Research Center for Independent Living, Ireland) by Senior Researcher Joseph Wherton; ambient-assisted living perspectives by Anssi Ylimaula, Vice CEO of Mawell Group, Oulu, Finland; and an overview of a commercial remote specialist diagnosis service that was presented by Timo Hakkarainen, the Managing Director of Remote Analysis (RemoteA) Ltd., Helsinki, Finland. HWTS 2011 ended with a summarizing panel discussion that brought vividly to front many hot topics encountered in the presentations and also generated interesting brainstorming for future directions of the field.

Our workshop would not have been possible without the support of the TPC members who dedicated time and effort to their reviews. The GPC conference organizers provided great support in ensuring the smooth running of the event! Further, the Academy of Finland MOTIVE program coordinators Anssi Mälkki and Mikko Ylikangas showed important dedication to our workshop, which also turned out to be an important platform for the interaction of researchers from closely related MOTIVE projects. We also thank the authors for their diligent efforts in writing, presenting and revising their papers, as well as Springer for publishing the proceedings.

May 2011

Timo O. Korhonen
Edward Mutafungwa

Organization

Conference Chairs

Timo Korhonen   Aalto University, Finland
Edward Mutafungwa   Aalto University, Finland

Technical Program Committee

Eija Kaasinen   Technical Research Centre of Finland, Finland
Hannele Hyppönen   National Institute for Health and Welfare,
                               Finland
Jari Aro   Tampere University, Finland
Jari Iinatti   Centre of Wireless Communication, Oulu,
                               Finland
Jiao Bingli   Peking University, China
Johanna Viitanen   Aalto University, Finland
Juha Röning   University of Oulu, Finland
Matti Hämäläinen   Aalto University, Finland
Minna Isomursu   Technical Research Centre of Finland, Finland
Olli Silven   University of Oulu, Finland
Pekka Ruotsalainen   National Institute for Health and Welfare,
                               Finland
Pirkko Nykänen   Tampere University, Finland
Qin Gao   Tsinghua University, China
Raimo Sepponen   Aalto University, Finland
Timo Itälä   Aalto University, Finland
Timo Jämsä   University of Oulu, Finland
Vesa Pakarinen   Technical Research Centre of Finland, Finland
Yuping Zhao   Peking University, China

External Reviewer

Iiro Jantunen   Aalto University, Finland

Doctoral Colloquium
Preface

The Doctoral Colloquium held in conjunction with the Grid and Pervasive Computing Conference had the same scope as the main conference. We invited PhD students and candidates to present, discuss and defend their work-in-progress or preliminary results with an international and renowned audience of researchers and developers. The Doctoral Colloquium aims at offering PhD students high-quality feedback from external reviewers and allowing them to directly interact with peers, to exchange ideas, discuss concepts, and establish informal cooperation between researchers and research groups.

PhD students and candidates at all stages in the process were invited to submit a thesis position paper, but preference was given to students early on in their PhD work. The call for thesis position papers was made public on the GPC 2011 website and by other channels. A review and selection was performed as a peer-review process that obeys the GPC 2011 conflict of interest policy. The Doctorial Colloquium Chairs and Panellists formed the Program Committee which reviewed and selected the papers. The authors were given feedback and an opportunity to revise the papers before the Doctorial Colloquium. The papers in these proceedings are the revised versions. The Doctorial Colloquium took place on May 10, 2011. Participants gave short, informal presentations of their work during the colloquium, which was followed by a discussion.

Seven PhD candidates submitted papers before the deadline and after the review all were accepted. As can be expected in a pervasive and grid computing conference, the topics of the papers had a wide scope and they represented different viewpoints and sub-disciplines within the ICT field. The topics included context-aware micro-architectures for smart spaces, frameworks for creating and evaluating persuasive games and applications; middleware for dynamic processing of sensor data; a concept for equipping smart spaces with metacognitive functionality; models for an inherently privacy-preserving ubiquitous application framework; new methods for creating mash-ups for mobile and fixed devices; and a light-weight architecture facilitating cooperation between applications. The wide spectrum of topics and approaches made the discussion in the Doctorial Colloquium most interesting and lively. It is our hope that the feedback and discussion helped the candidates with their work.

We would like to express our gratitude to the Program Committee members and panellistsJonnaHäkkilä, NatasaMilic-Frayling, and Jukka Riekki who gave their time and expertise and thus made the Doctorial Colloquium possible. Also, we thank the organizers of the GPC conference, both local and international. Finally, we thank and congratulate the PhD candidates for presenting – and defending – their most interesting work. Good luck in your pursuit!

Heikki Ailisto
Aaron Quigley

Doctoral Colloquium
Organization

Organizing Committee

Heikki Ailisto   VTT Technical Research Centre of Finland, Oulu, Finland

Aaron Quigley   The University of St. Andrews, Scotland, UK

Jonna Häkkilä   Nokia Research Center, Oulu, Finland

Natasa Milic-Frayling   Microsoft Research, Cambridge, UK

Jukka Riekki   University of Oulu, Finland

Table of Contents

International Workshop on Self-managing Solutions for Smart Environments (S3E 2011)

International Workshop on Health and Well-being Technologies and Services for Elderly (HWTS 2011)

Doctoral Colloquium

Global Understanding Environment:
Towards Self-managed Web of Everything

Vagan Terziyan

Industrial Ontologies Group
University of Jyväskylä, Finland
vagan.terziyan@jyu.fi

Abstract. Current Web grows rapidly to several directions (from the Web of Documents to the Webs of Humans, Things, Services, Knowledge, Intelligence, etc.). Consequently the recent and future Web-based applications, systems and frameworks (like, e.g., Social and Ubiquitous Computing, SOA and Cloud Computing, etc.) should take into account challenges related to extremely high heterogeneity of components and exponentially increased complexity of a business logic connecting and making them interoperable. Enabling self-management enhanced with semantic technology seems to be an only option to handle that. We suggest adding a "virtual representative" to every resource in the Web to solve the global interoperability problem. Intelligent agent (a kind of "software robot") will act, communicate and collaborate as a proxy on behalf of each Web resource. It will be connected with its resource via "semantic adapter", will communicate with other agents via "semantic communication" and will be coordinated via "semantic business logic". The relevant "Global Understanding Environment" (GUN) vision of Industrial Ontologies Group will be briefly presented. It can be considered as a kind of ubiquitous eco-system, which will be such proactive, self-managed evolutionary Semantic Web of Everything where all kinds of entities are assumed to understand, interact, serve, develop and learn from each other. The key set of enabling technologies for the GUN vision implementation includes: Artificial Intelligence; Semantic and Agent technologies; SOA and Cloud Computing. Some activities and projects, results and lessons learned by Industrial Ontologies Group on their way towards GUN will be briefly discussed.

Industrial Ontologies Group (IOG)

The IOG has been created in 2002 by initiative of international researchers and students from Agora Center and Department of Mathematical Information Technology in University of Jyvaskyla. The major concept developed by the group is "Global Understanding Environment" (GUN) and the major activities are related to the "Roadmap towards GUN". Among those there are: SmartResource project (2004-2007) - "Proactive Self-Maintained Resources in Semantic Web" funded by TEKES and investigating industrial applications of semantic and agent technologies; and more recent TEKES project called UBIWARE (2007-2010) - "Smart Semantic Middleware

M. Rautiainen et al. (Eds.): GPC 2011 Workshops, LNCS 7096, pp. 1–2, 2012.

for Ubiquitous Computing", in which a platform and a set of tools has been developed for creation and operation of self-managed complex industrial systems consisting of distributed, heterogeneous components of different nature. Currently the group takes part is the project within Cloud Software TIVIT (ICT-SHOK) Program, in which the group utilizes UBIWARE for various tasks within cloud environments.

Smart Solutions for Risk Prevention
through Analysis of People Movements

MariaGrazia Fugini[1], Stefano Pinardi[2], and Claudia Raibulet[2]

[1] Politecnico di Milano, Dipartimento di Elettronica e Informatica, Via Ponzio, 34/5,
20133, Milan, Italy
[2] Università degli Studi di Milano-Bicocca, Dipartimento di Informatica, Sistemistica e
Comunicazione, Viale Sarca 336, Ed. U14, 20126, Milan, Italy
fugini@elet.polimi.it, {pinardi,raibulet}@disco.unimib.it

Abstract. The high number of accidents in living areas, work environments, and
ambient, in general, can benefit of prevention mechanisms able to identify the
causes and the indications which precede accidents, and to put in place strategies
to avoid risks whenever this is possible. To this aim, this paper presents a risk
management architecture for monitoring movements within a smart ambient and
managing possible risks. In particular, we present a methodology for movement
analysis aimed at detecting and preventing risks. Results from experimentations
are discussed.

Keywords: risk, emergency, risk management, smart environments.

1 Introduction

One of the goals of a smart environment is to support and enhance the abilities of its
occupants in executing tasks. In particular, in living areas, work plants, or
construction environments, these tasks can present a high level of risk, ranging from
moving around in a (potentially dangerous) space to interacting with objects/machines
and handling (potentially dangerous) tools.

To support the occupants in facing possible risks, the concept of *smart
environment* is introduced along with concepts of self-healing features and ambient
intelligence [2, 15]. Sensors and devices can be distributed in the areas to detect the
current state (*context)* of the environment and determine what actions should be taken
to face or prevent risks (self-healing system) [5, 13, 19, 21]. The context consists of
any information that can be used to characterize the situation (or state) of an *entity*,
namely, a person, a place, a physical or computational object, or a machine, a tool, a
protection kit or a sensor network. This information can include personal movements,
physical gestures, relationships between persons and objects in the environment,
features of the physical environment such as spatial layout and temperature, and
identity the location of people and objects in the environment.

This paper proposes an approach to *location-based risk analysis* in combination
with a *movement recognition method*. To create a smart environment, where such an

M. Rautiainen et al. (Eds.): GPC 2011 Workshops, LNCS 7096, pp. 3–13, 2012.
© Springer-Verlag Berlin Heidelberg 2012

approach is possible, smart tags can be employed, such as sensors, RFID, or smart phones that can be carried or worn by persons to allow the detection of their location, their proximity to potentially dangerous sources and to determine the risk they are exposed to at a given instant. In particular, we propose a method enabling to detect what risks can possibly arise due *to the movements* of a person in the area. We focus on the use of *inertial sensors* for such monitoring. Inertial sensors are low cost devices that measure linear forces and torque forces, and which can be worn on body. These are becoming smaller and smaller, so increasing the user acceptance of body-worn sensors. Movement classification with inertial sensor showed to be useful in many areas like ambient intelligent and healthcare applications, in neuroscience and for tracking activities [1, 12, 15, 18]. Inertial sensors can also be used for human computer interaction, gait and posture analysis, and motion capture, or to understand emotional status from body posture [3, 10]. A large literature exists about the use of inertial sensors to classify movements, with different results. Many of the proposed methodologies are specific to problems or applications or to the given technology. Hence, sometimes they are hardly to translate into practice, or they use minimal dictionaries (3-6 actions), hence not allowing for the use of a method that could be reused in different contexts [1, 23]. Recently, a new technique called *Distributed Sparsity Classifier* has been proposed [23], where a public database of movements is introduced, called WARD 1.0, which has been made available and which we used to compare and test the results of our approach. Based on information we can obtain from inertial sensors, we define applications that use the context to provide task-relevant information and/or services to a user, hence to be context-aware [7]. In this paper, we show how information collected from the environment can be conveyed to a *Risk Management System* able to compute and re-distribute information signalling risks and emergencies, where emergencies are defined as situations that have a high danger and must be faced immediately. Risk is instead defined as a situation which evolves smoothly (such as a gas loss or a moving machine) which can be notified and prevented.

This paper is organized as follows. Section 2 introduces our architectural perspective to risk management. Section 3 presents how movements in our application domain are monitored and the methodology for movement analysis, with tests and results and ICS and ECS (intra cluster inter cluster) measures. Section 4 presents a sample scenario. Conclusions and further work are given in Section 5.

2   An Architectural Perspective towards Risks

Our *Risk Management System* (*RMS*) (see Figure 1) exploits the Monitoring, Analyzing, Planning, Executing (MAPE) loop [6, 11]. This loop observes the environment, detects the anomalies by analyzing the data collected through the monitoring step, decides if a risky situation occurred and if intervention/change is needed and of what type, and puts in place (executes) the planned modifications in the environment. The main tasks of the MAPE risk control loop are:

1) *Monitoring* is continuously performed through a set of sensors (e.g., RFID sensors, video cameras, inertial sensors) and devices (e.g., PDAs, PCs) called here *informative devices*. Such devices are distributed in the environment (e.g., on the machines/tools, on the persons and on equipment) and collect data regarding for example the level of gas, the movement of machineries and persons, the operations performed using a tool (e.g., a hammer, a water container), or the health conditions of persons.

2) *Analysis* on the monitored data verifies if data are out of ordinary values (e.g., the gas level is >= a threshold, or a machinery is moving towards an area where persons are working, the hearth pressure of a person is in the normal range).
   A threshold is a point value or a range which delimitates regions of risks from the normal/ordinary values. If the *Risk Threshold* is respected, the system operates normally. In between the *Risk* and the *Emergency Threshold*, the system is operating in a risky status, where preventive actions can still be put in place to prevent the risk. Beyond the *Emergency Threshold*, the system operates in *emergency* [8], and corrective actions are applied.

3) *Planning* is performed when in one (or more) monitored element is out of the admitted ranges. In the planning, our solution associates a risk evaluation function to each element in the environment. By combining all the risks evaluations, we determine if we are in face of a risk, an emergency, or a false alarm. In case of risk, in the planning, the *RMS* selects the most suitable strategy (a set of interventions) able to reduce or eliminate the risk.

4) *Executing* applies the strategies identified in the planning phase. Upon application of the strategies, the loop continues with the monitoring phase.

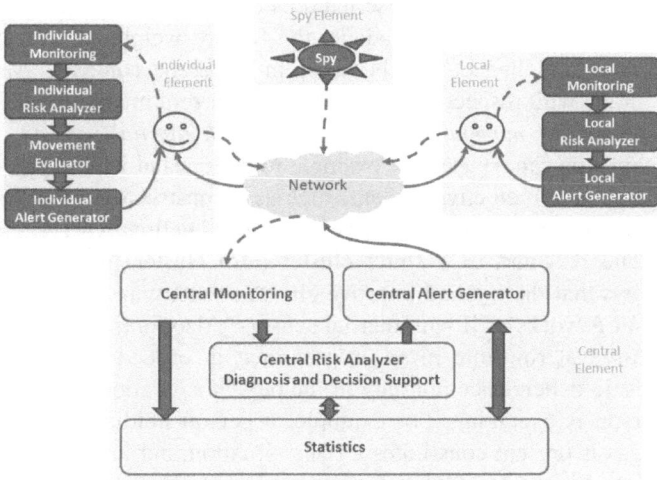

Fig. 1. Risk Management Architecture

The risk model supported by the architecture shown in Figure 1 is based on modeling explicitly both risk and environment entities meaningful for risk computation [7, 8]. In particular, the risk model is person centred, in that it relates the risk to the user behaviour and movements (work activities in our case study). We have presented our approach in [7, 8, 9]. In this paper, we deal with *monitoring the persons' activities* using body-worn informative devices (see next sections).

3   Monitoring Persons' Movements

There are many specific advantages in using body-worn sensors instead of video cameras for movement classification. Inertial sensors can be placed on specific segments of the body or in clothes accessories. Consequently, we know with absolute certainty which segment of the body the data refers to, and we do not have to solve "hidden parts" problems, nor solve color and luminance issues typical of video cameras. Also, we do not have to segment the body from the other environment information, or to disambiguate and interpret data when many people are present in the same area [4, 14, 17]. On the other hand, there is no general methodology to classify movements that can be used in different situations or with different technologies. The usual approaches are very specific to the given situation. After an accurate study of the Dictionary of actions [16, 20], very specific features are chosen and used. When we change the Dictionary, the recognition accuracy is not guaranteed.

In this paper, we show why the method of *FFxIVFF* significantly improves accuracy of movement classification by using inertial sensors. The method exploits a procedure, called *FFxIVFF*, which automatically changes the movement features weighting in function of the movements [16, 20]. *FFxIVFF* transforms the space, lowering, in the Dictionary, the importance of those features that are less discriminative, and incrementing those features that are more frequent within a given class. The procedure automatically adapts the feature weighting with respect to the given Dictionary, and hence, can be used in different contexts. Also, it greatly improves accuracy with respect to other recent concurrent methodologies, providing a general instrument for *movement classification with inertial sensors*. A movement classifier of this type can be used for example to understand which type of actions are executed by a person in an environment, such as a construction plant or an industrial area where there are people at work, given a proper Dictionary of actions as showed in [16, 20]. The ICS and ECS (inter cluster intra cluster) measures, given in the Section 3, shows that the method improve clusters density and separation, explaining why the *FFxIVFF* works well with inertial sensors. Also, in this research, this kind of classifiers is used at run-time in an environment in order to understand if a risky situation arises, in dependence not only of the person's location but specifically of the action the person is executing. For example, a person holding a lighter where free inflammable gas is present constitutes a risky situation, but until the lighter is off the risk is relatively low. An actual risk arises when a person tries to ignite it in the environment. A *movement classifier* with inertial sensors can understand this kind of risky situation, which depends on the person's actions and on the situation, and can help avoiding it. The benefits of intervening in such risky circumstances and avoid catastrophic situations are evident.

3.1   Methodology for Movement Classification

For movement analysis, we used five MTx inertial sensors of XSens [22]. Each MTx sensor has three components: an accelerometer, a gyroscope, and a magnetometer with three degrees of freedom, providing information on acceleration (+/- 50 m/sec2), rate of turn (+/-2 rad/sec), and earth-magnetic field (+/-1 normalized) in a three-axial reference system. In order to recognize a movement, we need a *database of movements* to create our test set and to generate the *FFxIVFF* [16, 20]. Consequently, a specific set of actions is executed by a set of people and features are extracted from the generated data, action by action, sample by sample using an iterative procedure. In order to obtain these data, we employ a tool which simulates data transmission from sensors (details are presented in [9]). In particular, each component – accelerometer, gyroscope, and magnetometer – has three dimensional data (X,Y,Z). Every datum is also considered in its 2D and 3D norm representation (|XY|, |XZ|, |YZ|, |XYZ|). Then, data are filtered using eight transformation functions (null, smoothing, low pass, mean, variance, variance with low pass, first derivative, second derivative) generating 840 different signals from the original ones. These transformation functions are very generic, and are quite common in the movement classification area. Then, for each transformation 10 generic features are chosen generating 8400 features. Feature values are quantized into 22 intervals for a total of 184.800 intervals: when hit a specific interval is marked 1, otherwise is left to 0. Hence, every action generates a sparse vector of 184.800 binary values. The given values are stored in a vector. Values are quantized, and *FF* and *IVFF* are calculated. Hence, any action is transformed into a *n*-dimensional vector in a *n*-dimensional Feature-Action space. The set of quantized features-action vectors of an action executed by a population and reweighted by *FFxIVFF* constitutes the pattern of the given type of action. When a new action is executed, we transform it (using a run-time procedure) into a vector of the Feature-Action space using the same methodology. Then, we calculate how similar it is to the given type of actions, using a similarity measure. In particular we use three popular similarity measures: a Ranking algorithm (Eq.1), an Euclidean Distance (Eq.2), and a Cosine Similarity (Eq.3). The formulas are the following:

$$\text{rank}_j = \sum_{i=1}^{n} W_{i,j} \qquad (1)$$

$$\text{dist}_i = \sqrt{\sum_{j=1}^{n} \left(W_{i,j} - q_{i,j} \right)^2} \qquad (2)$$

$$\cos \theta = \frac{W_{i,j} \cdot q_{i,j}}{|W_{i,j}||q_{i,j}|} \qquad (3)$$

where $W_{i,j}$ represents the weight of the σ_i interval of action a_j of the Training-Set, and $q_{i,j}$ is the IVFF value associated to the feature of query.

3.2   The *FFxIVFF* Transformation

In this space, the centroids of the actions cluster are too close to each other, making the recognition a problem. In order to increase the accuracy, and use algorithms that are fast and feasible in run-time applications but are still reliable in term of accuracy, we transform the feature action space into a different space by appropriately reweighting the features values (see [15, 16]). Hence, two weights have been introduced: the *FF* ("Feature Frequency") and the *IVFF* ("Inverse vocabulary frequency"). The *FF* formula:

$$FF_{i,j} = \frac{n_{i,j}}{|P|} \tag{4}$$

where $n_{i,j}$ is the number of occurrences of the σ_i feature in the action a_j, and $|P|$ represents the population cardinality. The *IVFF* formula is:

$$IVFF_i = \log \frac{|A|}{|\{a : \sigma_i \in a\}|} \tag{5}$$

where $|A|$ represents the cardinality of the vocabulary, and $|\{a : \sigma_i \in a\}|$ the number of actions a where feature σ_i assumes values. The overall weight of a single feature is given by the multiplication: $W_{i,j} = FF_{i,j} * IVFF_i$. The *FF* takes into account how frequent is a feature in the given population rising the importance of the features that appear in the same class of movements (Eq.4). The *IVFF* takes into account how frequent is a feature in the dictionary: a feature that is present in more actions is considered less discriminative, and its weight is lowered according to the formula (Eq. 5.). We note that the *FFxIVFF* space is different from the original values space: some dimensions can be canceled or enhanced depending on the role of features in the dictionary and population. The *FFxIVFF* transforms the original space into a space where clusters appear to be denser and more separated. This approach allows reaching high accuracy (the highest in literature as far as we know), using very simple and fast algorithms of similarity.

3.3   The Datasets

In order to test the proposed method, we used two databases: NIDA 1.0 (Nomadis internal Database of Actions) the database of the Nomadis Laboratory at the University of Milano-Bicocca (see [20]) and the WARD 1.0 (Wearable Action Recognition Database) created at UC Berkeley [23]. These databases are quite representative of a typical database of actions, since they are large (respectively 273 and 1200 samples) and have a large number of actions (respectively, 13 and 21). They are quite different for issues such as sensors technology, dimension of the vocabulary of actions, number and type of samples, and granularity of low level data. NIDA 1.0 contains 21 types of actions for a total of 273 samples. These actions are:

> 1. Get up from seat. 2. Get up from a chair. 3. Open a wardrobe. 4. Open a door. 5. Fall. 6. Walk forward 7. Run. 8. Turn left 180 degrees. 9. Turn right 180 degrees. 10. Turn left 90 degrees. 11. Turn right 90 degrees. 12. Karate frontal kick. 13. Karate side kick. 14. Karate punch. 15. Go upstairs. 16. Go downstairs. 17. Jump. 18. Write. 19. Lie down on a seat. 20. Sitting on a chair. 21. Heavily sitting on a chair.

WARD contains 13 types of actions performed by 20 people ranging from 20 to 79-years-old with 5 repetition per action, for a total of 1200 actions. The list of actions is the following:

1. Stand (ST). 2. Sit (SI). 3. Lie down (LI). 4. Walk forward (WF). 5. Walk left-circle (WL). 6. Walk right circle (WR). 7. Turn left (TL). 8. Turn right (TR). 9. Go upstairs (UP). 10. Go downstairs (DO). 11. Jog (JO). 12. Jump (JU). 13. Drive truck (PU).

3.4   Tests and Results

Even if the two databases are technologically different, the methodology has been applied – as is – without significant changes to both the databases, using a Leave One Out Cross Validation (LOOCV) methodology. Recognition accuracies are very high in both cases. The classification accuracies using the NIDA 1.0 database (273 samples of 21 type actions) are the followings: Ranking 89.74%, Euclidean Distance 95.23%, Cosine similarity 95.23%. The classification accuracies of algorithms using the WARD 1.0 database are the followings: Ranking 97.5%, Euclidean Distance 97.74%, Cosine 97.63%. We have to note that the accuracy of our methodology applied to the WARD 1.0 database outperforms their results [see 23]. The UC Berkeley researchers reached and accuracy of only 93.4 % using their databases. In particular, we reduced by three times the error rate (from 6.6% to 2.26%).

Other tests have been done to test the accuracy reducing the number of worn sensors, to check the sensitivity to sensor numbers [16]. Using WARD 1.0 with 3 sensors on the pelvis, the right wrist, and ankle, we reached an accuracy of 97.63% (with the cosine similarity), and using only one sensor we reached a 93.62% of accuracy (with cosine similarity), against the 93.4 % of U.C. Berkeley obtained on the same database with *all* the 5 sensors.

In order to understand why the proposed method has far better accuracy than former methodologies, we tried to understand which effects *FFxIVFF* has on dimension of clusters both in WARD 1.0 and NIDA 1.0 multidimensional spaces.

At this aim, the Intracluster (ICS) and Intercluster (ECS) have been calculated, and measures confirm that the *FFxIVFF* creates a space where clusters are more dense and well separated, justifying the higher accuracies obtained in the tests sections with the LOOCV methodology. Intracluster and Intercluster similarity have been measured in the values space, then in the *FF* space and finally in the *FFxIVFF* space. Cosine similarity has been used as a similarity measure. Results have been compared and showed in Table 1.

Note that *FF* and *IVFF* actually enhance cluster density and cluster separation, respectively. In particular, using the NIDA database, we can note that:

- *IVFF* enhances the Intercluster similarity 5.96 times wrt *FF*, and 12.23 times wrt the values space;
- *FF* enhances the Intracluster similarity, while thanks to *FFxIVFF* Intracluster similarity passes the critical threshold of 0.9.

While using WARD database we can note that:

- *IVFF* enhances the Intercluster similarity 4.08 times wrt the values space
- *FF* enhances the Intracluster similarity, while thanks to *FFxIVFF* Intracluster similarity passes the critical threshold of 0.9.

The Intracluster and Intercluster similarity confirm us the reasons why *FFxIVFF* works well. Clusters are more dense and further apart (the values of Intercluster similarity has been improved of one order), significantly reducing the probability of false positives. Thanks to that, it is possible to classify movements with greater accuracy even using a few sensors (three). Note that it is possible to recognize movements that involve parts of body that have not a sensor placed on it. The accuracy results, confirmed by ICS and ECS measures, sustains the idea that the *FFxIVFF* methodology is solid, and allow us to propose the use of this methodology in actual situations, even at runtime.

Table 1. Intracluster similarity before and after *FFxIVFF*

Database	Type	Value Space (Cos)	FF space (Cos)	FFxIVFF space (Cos)
Nida	Intercluster	0,3506425	0,1710151	0,0286604
	Intracluster	0,7077682	0,8759209	0,9260479
Ward	Intercluster	0,2476419	0,2367639	0,0605941
	Intracluster	0,6038969	0,8455223	0,9311265

The independence of technology, the possibility to use few sensors, and the feasibility of these results confirmed by the ICS and ECS measure, give us now the scientific ground for a real use of the method. In this case, we propose to use three body worn sensors, to understand which kind of movements has been executed, and to relate risk analysis to movements, as we can see in the next section.

4   Movements' Analysis in Risk Management: A Sample Scenario

In work areas, users employ tools or drive machines. We only examine risk related to movements of persons in handling these tools and machines (namely, we ignore the case of risks *generated* by tools and machines). We can monitor the persons' movements and check the risk which they are exposed to. We assume that inertial sensors are worn by persons and allow risk to be identified by the *Movement Evaluator* module of the Risk Management Architecture. We assume that other sensors, e.g., RFID for determining the location of the various entities - objects, persons - in the environment, are in place to detect other risks. Based on these affirmations, we are currently extending the database of actions with work specific activities. We associate a Risk Level to each work related action in the range [0..5] where risk increases from 0 to 5. Examples of clusters of actions bound to their Risk Levels will include:

1. Enter work area. 2. Go upstairs at the second floor. 3. Use hammer. 4. Turn left 90 degrees. 5. Stop working. 6. Go downstairs. 7. Leave the work area.

Risk Level = 3

1. Enter work area. 2. Step into the truck. 3. Drive the truck. 4. Stop the truck. 5. Leave the area.

Risk Level = 5

The Movement Evaluator module of our architecture (see Figure 1) performs a continuous monitoring of the persons/tools and machinery through both identifications (e.g., RFID) obtained by applying passive tags on instruments and inertial sensors. Through controlled points in the environment, the system is aware of which tool a worker is interacting with at a given moment and hence, executes given check operations. A catalogue of all work tools and their assignment to workers is available. The Movement Evaluator determines if a person is at risk by using a *RiskEvaluation* function. Such function analyses the parameters characterizing each person/tool and machinery interaction by: a) evaluating the data retrieved from the sensors; b) correlating such data to the Risk Level assigned to actions. The trend of the *RiskEvaluation* function is defined by a utility function: e.g., linear, logarithmic, exponential, sigmoid. We assume that the output of an evaluation is normalized and always included in [0..1]. Namely, we have:

$$evaluation\_value = f\,(parameter)$$

where f denotes the evaluation function and parameter represents the elements monitored to determine the risk, in this case the actions the person is performing with which tool and machinery. The *evaluation_value* is numeric and expresses the risk for each parameter. If it is beyond a given value (fixed for that particular parameter), a potential risk is signaled. For example, for the "closeness to moving crane", the lowest value corresponds to the best quality, while the highest value corresponds to a risk event. In our approach, a set of function f are stored in the *Movement Evaluator* files. There may be more parameters for one entity (e.g., tools/machineries, persons, protection garments, informative device). Depending on the risky situation, there may be various solutions for their management. For example, a worker is notified about his position to close to the location of a truck in movement or can receive a warning when walking forward in the direction of a dangerous machine. He is then required to use another type of tool or to adopt another strategy to achieve the same objective/task. These solutions are called *strategies* and are defined as sequences of actions to be executed with different priorities depending on the evaluated Risk Level. We have implemented a sample preliminary set of strategies in a prototype which is described in [9].

5   Concluding Remarks

In this paper we have presented an overview of our approach to risk management in smart environments based on the analysis of persons' movements. We have provided details on the method we adopt concerning the computation of persons' movements in the environment. From the architectural point of view, our solution exploits self-healing mechanisms by implementing the MAPE loop. Currently, our prototype for risk management addresses risks exploiting this loop. Its design allows the evolution towards the consideration of the detailed persons' movements, which we plan to integrate in the prototype in the next future.

Acknowledgments. This work has been partially supported by the TeKNE Project and by the S-Cube European Network of Excellence in Software Services and Systems.

References

1. Bao, L.: Physical Activity Recognition from Acceleration, Department of Electrical Engineering and Computer at the Massachusetts Institute of Technology, Master Thesis (August 2003)
2. Botts, M., Percivall, G., Reed, C., Davidson, J.: OGC® Sensor Web Enablement: Overview and High Level Architecture. In: Nittel, S., Labrinidis, A., Stefanidis, A. (eds.) GSN 2006. LNCS, vol. 4540, pp. 175–190. Springer, Heidelberg (2008)
3. Castellano, G., Villalba, S.D., Camurri, A.: Recognising Human Emotions from Body Movement and Gesture Dynamics. In: Paiva, A.C.R., Prada, R., Picard, R.W. (eds.) ACII 2007. LNCS, vol. 4738, pp. 71–82. Springer, Heidelberg (2007)
4. Cameron, J., Lasenby, J.: Estimating Human Skeleton Parameters and Configuration in Real-Time from Markered Optical Motion Capture. In: Proceedings of the 5th International Conference on Articulated Motion and Deformable Objects (2008)
5. Chen, N., Di, L., Yu, G., Min, M.: A Flexible Geospatial Sensor Observation Service for Diverse Sensor Data based on Web Service. ISPRS Journal of Photogrammetry and Remote Sensing 64, 234–242 (2009)
6. Cheng, B.H.C., de Lemos, R., Giese, H., Inverardi, P., Magee, J.: Software Engineering for Self-Adaptive Systems. LNCS, vol. 5525. Springer, Heidelberg (2009)
7. Conti, G.M., Rizzo, F., Fugini, M.G., Raibulet, C., Ubezio, L.: Wearable Services in Risk Management. In: IEEE/WIC/ACM International Joint Conferences on Web Intelligence and Intelligent Agent Technologies, Web2Touch Workshop, pp. 563–566 (2009)
8. Fugini, M.G., Raibulet, C., Ubezio, L.: Risk Characterization and Prototyping. In: Proceedings of the 10th International Conference on New Technologies of Distributed Systems (NOTERE 2010), Tozeur, Tunisia, May 31-June 2, pp. 57–64 (2010)
9. Fugini, M.G., Raibulet, C., Ramoni, F.: Service-Oriented Architecture for Risk Management. In: Proc. 11th Int. Conf. on New Technologies of Distributed Systems, NOTERE 2011, Paris, May 10-12 (2011)
10. Kleinsmith, A., Bianchi-Berthouze, N.: Recognizing affective dimensions from body posture. In: Paiva, A.C.R., Prada, R., Picard, R.W. (eds.) ACII 2007. LNCS, vol. 4738, pp. 48–58. Springer, Heidelberg (2007)
11. Laguna, M.A., Finat, J., González, J.A.: Mobile health monitoring and smart sensors: a product line approach. In: Proceedings of the 2009 Euro American Conference on Telematics and Information Systems: New Opportunities To increase Digital Citizenship (EATIS 2009), pp. 1–8. ACM, New York (2009)
12. Lee, S., Mase, K.: Activity and Location Recognition using Wearable Sensors. IEEE Pervasive Computing, 24–32 (2002)

13. Lundgren, R.E., McMakin, A.H.: Risk Communication. In: A Handbook for Communicating Environmental, Safety, and Health Risks, 4th edn., Wiley Publ. (2009)
14. Moeslund, T.B., Granum, E.: A Survey of Computer Vision-Based Human Motion Capture. Computer Vision and Image Understanding (2001)
15. Mileo, A., Merico, D., Pinardi, S., Bisiani, R.: A Logical Approach to Home Healthcare with Intelligent Sensor-Network Support. The Computer Journal (2009)
16. Mileo, A., Pinardi, S., Bisiani, R.: Movement Recognition using Context: a Lexical Approach based on Coherence. In: Proceedings of the Sixth International Workshop on Modeling and Reasoning in Context (2010)
17. Okada, R., Stenger, B.: A Single Camera Motion Capture System for Human-Computer Interaction. IEEE Transactions on Information and Systems E91-D(7), 1855–1862 (2008)
18. Ohgi, S., Morita, S., Loo, K.K., Mizuike, C.: Time Series Analysis of Spontaneous Upper-Extremity Movements of Premature Infants With Brain Injuries. Phys. Ther. 88(9), 1022–1033 (2008)
19. Pederson, T., Surie, D.: Towards an Activity-Aware Wearable Computing Platform Based on an Egocentric Interaction Model. In: Ichikawa, H., Cho, W.-D., Chen, Y., Youn, H.Y. (eds.) UCS 2007. LNCS, vol. 4836, pp. 211–227. Springer, Heidelberg (2007)
20. Pinardi, S., Bisiani, B.: Movement Recognition with Intelligent Multisensor Analysis, a Lexical Approach. In: Workshops Proceedings of the 6th International Conference on Intelligent Environments, pp. 170–177 (2010)
21. Rubio, J., Padillo, I., Espina, J., Verástegui, J., López-de-Ipiña, J.: RFID in workplace safety solutions in Proceedings RFID Systech 2010. In: European Workshop on Smart Objects: Systems, Technologies and Applications, Ciudad, Spain, June 15-16 (2010)
22. XSens, http://www.xsens.com
23. Yang, A.Y., Jafari, R., Sastry, S.S., Bajcsy, R.: Distributed Recognition of Human Actions Using Wearable Motion Sensor Networks. Journal of Ambient Intelligence and Smart Environments (2009)

Supporting Situation-Awareness in Smart Spaces

Susanna Pantsar-Syväniemi, Jarkko Kuusijärvi, and Eila Ovaska

VTT Technical Research Centre of Finland,
Kaitoväylä 1,
90571 Oulu, Finland
{Susanna.Pantsar-Syvaniemi,Jarkko.Kuusijarvi,
Eila.Ovaska}@vtt.fi

Abstract. This paper reports results from ongoing research, relating to the development of the context ontology described with web ontology language (OWL). Our aim is to reach relevant context ontology for smart spaces that are, by their very nature, heterogeneous, pervasive and ubiquitous. We illustrate the usage of the context ontology in a case where lights are switched on according to a calculated wake-up time and the preferences of an individual. With the introduced Context Ontology for Smart Spaces, CO4SS, we managed to perform reasoning actions based on the user's context.

1   Introduction

A smart space is an environment that provides services to the inhabitants and visitors, according to, e.g., their situations and available communication capabilities. Hence, the smart space is an information-driven environment, where physical objects consume and provide digital information. The ability to take into account the context of the user, and the digital and physical environment makes a space smart. With the help of context information, the smart space application can be context-aware and react to the current situations or be proactive and take future circumstances into account. The context ontology is used as a common language in the smart spaces, to store and recognize the different context information and to enable this information to be used at run-time.

It is challenging to create convenient, general and relevant concepts for the context ontology that is suitable for the heterogeneous smart spaces. Hence, there are no recent results relating to these kinds of context ontologies. Although the context ontology language (CoOL) [1], context broker architecture (CoBrA) [2], service-oriented context-aware middleware (SOCAM) [3], context management ontology (COMANTO) [4], and a standard ontology for ubiquitous and pervasive applications (SOUPA) [5] are a few years old and applied to service oriented systems in different application domains, rather little emphasis has been placed on services, including their functional properties and related aspects, such as user interfaces and devices on which these services are deployed, along with temporal contextual information [6]. Furthermore, no attempts have been made to align service and context ontologies.

M. Rautiainen et al. (Eds.): GPC 2011 Workshops, LNCS 7096, pp. 14–23, 2012.

In the smart space, interactions are based on shared information and it is challenging to model and manage information coming from different sources as it can not be predefined and it is heterogeneous. Due to the inherent complexity of context-aware applications, the development should be supported by adequate context information modeling and reasoning techniques [7]. In [8] the authors point out that the development of context-aware applications is complex, as there are a large number of software engineering challenges stemming from, e.g., the heterogeneity of context information sources and the imperfection of context information.

This paper presents novel context ontology, CO4SS, and how it is formulated. We also illustrate the usage of the Context Ontology for Smart Spaces (CO4SS) in a case where lights are switched on according to a calculated wake-up time and the preferences of a person. We selected the ontology-based modeling approach and an OWL (Web Ontology Language) [9] for describing the context ontology. OWL supports the interoperability and heterogeneity that are needed for the ontology to be able to evolve in the future. Our context ontology, CO4SS, exploits some parts of the upper context conceptualization presented in [10].

The structure of the paper is as follows. Section 2 presents the background. Section 3 introduces our context ontology for smart spaces (CO4SS). Thereafter, Section 4 goes through the validation. Section 5 discusses our context ontology. Conclusions and future work close the paper.

2   Background

The highly used definition for context is: 'Context is any information that can be used to characterize the situation of an entity. An entity is a person, place, or object that is considered relevant to the interaction between a user and an application, including the user and applications themselves' [11]. In our earlier work, as introduced in [12], we proposed that 'A context defines the limit of the information usage of a smart space application'. This is based on the assumption that any piece of data, at a given time, can be context for a given smart space application.

The work presented here has its basis in a context-awareness concept that is our earlier work [13], where the conceptual context ontology is defined with three contextual levels: a physical context of the environment, a digital context of the environment and a situation context. The conceptual context ontology also has three contextual dimensions: physical (the changing (sensor) data of the execution environment), digital (context data derived from the physical data and state data of software artifacts) and a human, (a user with preferences and needs). Our context ontology is based on the semantic context information triangle presented in [7]. In addition to the conceptual context ontology, the context-awareness concept includes agents for context monitoring, reasoning and context-based adaptation. Thus, we have enhanced the concept of context-aware agents, presented as a context-aware micro-architecture in [14].

Our validation case, the adjustment of lighting according to a wake-up time and the preferences of an individual in the smart home, is designed according to an interoperability platform (IOP), developed in the SOFIA-project [15]. The purpose of the IOP is to make the information available between heterogeneous smart objects

(devices) and add semantics to this information. In the IOP, a SIB (Semantic Information Broker) creates a backbone for the smart space. In the SIB, all of the information
is based upon the idea of making statements in the form of subject-predicate-object
expressions. These expressions are known as triples in the Resource Description
Framework (RDF) [16]. A KP works as an independent agent, producing information
to and/or consuming it from the SIB. Thus, all of the information is transmitted via
the SIB, i.e., KPs do not communicate directly with each other. The information
transmission is performed by a SSAP (Smart Space Application Protocol). The SSAP
can be utilized with different communication protocols, e.g., TCP/IP and Bluetooth.
For the implementation, we utilized the RDF Information Base Solution (RIBS) [17]
which is one realization of the SIB defined in the IOP.

3   Context Ontology for Smart Spaces, CO4SS

In this section, we introduce the context ontology that we have developed incrementally and side by side with the context-awareness micro-architecture [14]. Our context
ontology i) conforms to the context-awareness micro-architecture developed for the
smart spaces, and ii) supports context-awareness and applications interoperability.
Our aim with the context ontology is to tackle the context modeling challenge when
the context information is as heterogeneous as it is in the smart spaces. Moreover, the
initial conceptual context ontology introduced in [13] has been enhanced to reach
wider and richer ontology in terms of concepts and properties. The initial context
ontology has been enhanced i) by separating the user context and the situational context, ii) by adding the social context, and iii) by defining each context dimension in
more detail. We discovered the need to expand our context ontology with the social
context during a case study where we developed a context-aware supervision of a
smart maintenance process [18]. Hence, our context ontology has five levels: physical, digital, situational, user, and social context, as illustrated in Fig. 1.

User context was separated from the Situational context because there is a need
to describe the user's context, preferences, etc., separately from the underlying

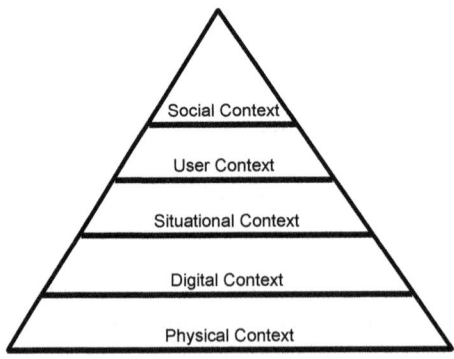

Fig. 1. The contextual levels of information in the context ontology, CO4SS

situations. Users have individual preferences and activities, which are both vital information for context-aware applications that serve the user. Furthermore, we wanted to modularize our ontology even more, thus, avoiding large OWL files, which would be hard to manage and update. Next, we will introduce the main concepts of these five levels with the help of ontology graphs.

The main class in our context ontology is *Context,* which has the following properties: state, time, and location. The *Context* has six subclasses, as shown in Fig. 2. Those classes are *Physical, Digital, Situational, User, Social,* and *Historical.* The SmartSpaceContext is, at least, composed of the Physical Context of the smart environment and the Digital Context of the smart environment. In addition, the User Context, Social Context, Historical Context, and the Situational Context can be part of the SmartSpaceContext. The properties of the Context are passed down to the subclasses of the SmartSpaceContext.

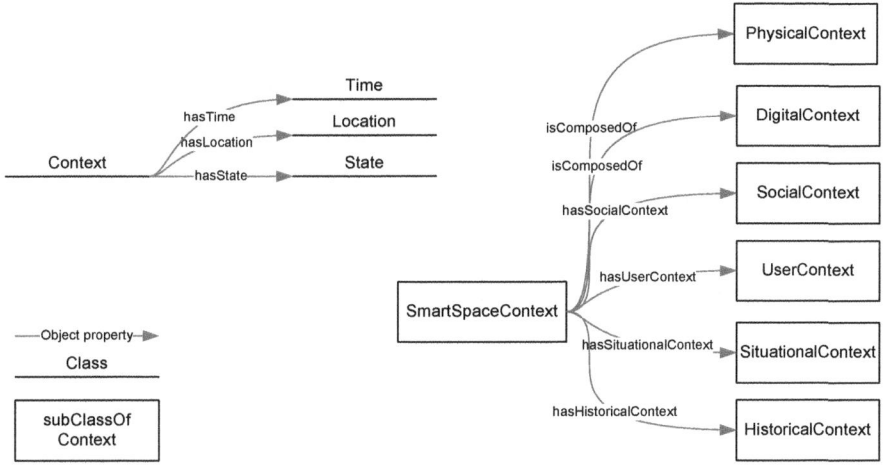

Fig. 2. The main class, *Context,* with its properties and subclasses

The *Physical* Context, presented in Fig. 3, describes the information coming from the physical and real objects, such as sensors. The Physical Context has active and passive objects, where the passive objects are more static and less capable than the active ones. We refer to the processing, communication and mobility capabilities. The Physical Context also represents real events that will happen in the smart spaces. The real events can be, e.g., output values coming from the sensors or devices, location updates, failures or connections made by objects that have arrived (or been added) to the smart space. The preferences of the users are saved to their smart spaces via devices. The events relate to the Situational Context. The adaptation in the smart space application is mostly triggered by the events.

The *Digital* Context, presented in Fig. 4, describes the information related to digital artifacts, e.g., features, services, applications. The Digital Context represents more inferred information that what is presented by the Physical Context. The Digital Context consists of agents, the features and rules, and the feature is respectively formed from the services and qualities. The features provide either one service or many services, i.e., a feature is a package of the services. The rules define the situations, i.e., the behavior of the (smart space) application. The services are specified with a unique service identification (ID) number, a description, and quality properties. The rules are specified by an identification (ID) number, a description, a target, and a value.

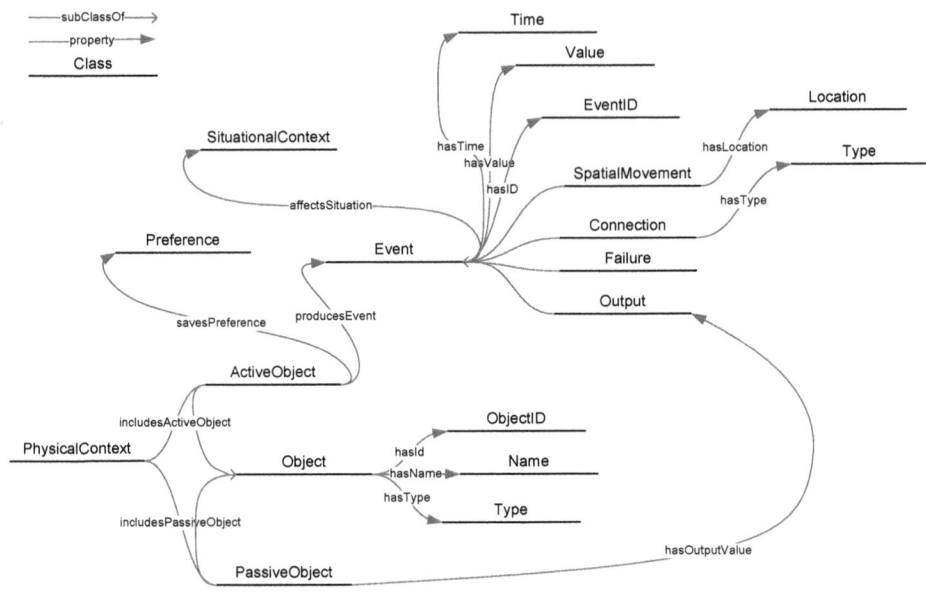

Fig. 3. The *Physical* context, with its properties and relations

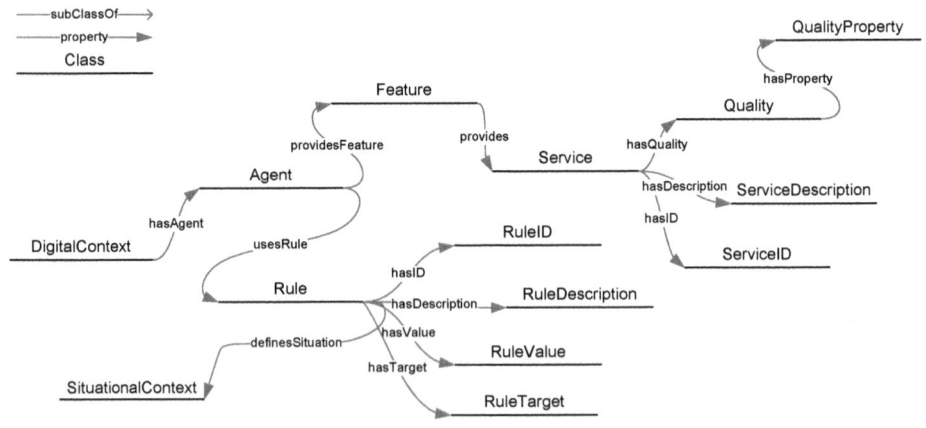

Fig. 4. The *Digital* context, with its properties and relations

The *Situational* Context has a description and identification (ID) number to help distinguish the situations from each other. The situations are affected by the preferences of the users and the social groups. The situations are defined by the rules and influenced by the events. The Situational Context is shown is Fig. 5.

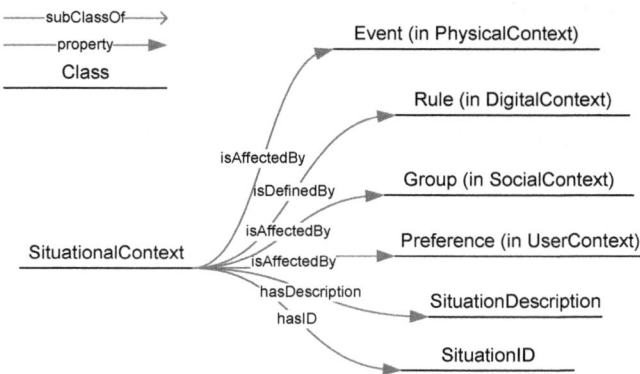

Fig. 5. The *Situational* context, with its properties and relations

The *User* Context defines a person with roles, preferences and friends, as presented in Fig. 6. For the details of the person and the group, we will use FOAF ontology [19]. The user affects the situations and belongs to the group(s). We included the Activity class to represent different kinds of activities, e.g., morning activities (showering, breakfast, morning newspapers, etc.), travel activities (work related travels, holiday travels, etc.), exercise activities (jogging, the gym, different games, etc.). These activities can be stored and used later on to make reasonings, according to different situations, e.g., how long does it usually take to perform morning activities.

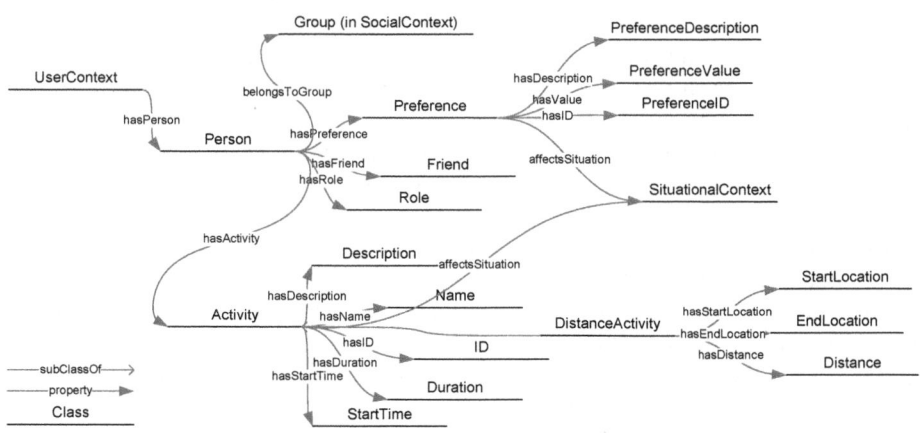

Fig. 6. The *User* Context, with its properties

The *Social* Context defines a group with properties and highlights that the group consists of persons. The group also affects the situations. The group also has its goal and positions. The Social context is illustrated in Fig. 7.

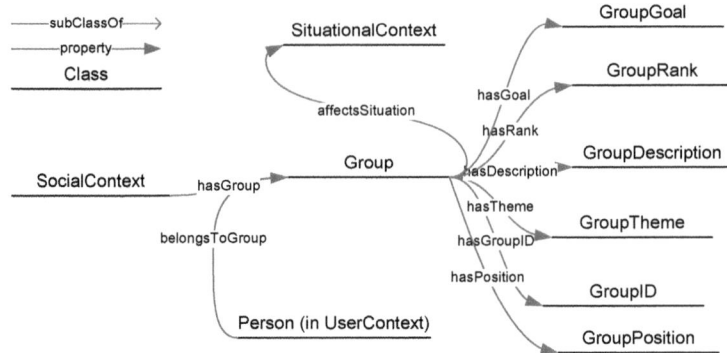

Fig. 7. The *Social* context, with its properties

4   Validation

We validated the context ontology with a scenario: the adjustment of lighting according to the wake-up time and the preferences of an individual in the smart home. The scenario is located in the personal smart space and combined with the person's smart home. The wake-up time is utilized from the SIB of the personal smart space and the preferences are consumed from the SIB of the smart home. Usually, only one SIB is utilized in an ordinary smart space application, but in this case, we consumed context information from two SIBs. We implemented the agents which were used in this case with the Python programming language and utilized RIBS [17] as the SIB for both the home and personal space. The aim of this validation was to discover whether context ontology is useful for reasoning actions based on the user's context.

The reasoning agent, running on the user's device, adds the user's preferences to his/her smart home. It also takes care of waking the user up at the correct time in the morning, as he/she wants. For example, if the user has a meeting in the morning, the application wakes the user up, so that he/she has time to do his/her morning activities and drive to the meeting place. The application utilizes the user's context information to find out how much time he/she uses for the morning activities, and finds out how much time it takes to drive to the meeting location (with a service that discovers the travel time from one place to another by a given transportation).

The reasoning agent, running on the smart home, takes care of everything which is related to the smart home. For example, it adjusts the lights according to the user's preferences at the time that he/she wants to wake-up. It could also adjust other home devices, according to the user's preferences.

We created a domain specific ontology for controlling the lighting in the user's home. Relevant parts of our context ontology were instantiated to be able to control and monitor the user's context. This validation scenario used the *Physical* Context class to describe the user's device that saves the preferences. Later on, the *DistanceActivity* could be used to provide historical information for the travel time, but it was not used in this scenario.

Digital Context described the reasoning *Agent* running on the home space, which provides the *Service* that wakes the user up, according to his/her preferences and wakeup-time. A *Rule* was instantiated to describe the actions that the *Agent* makes, although, at this time, this was merely a description, since dynamic *Rules* were not used. *Situational* Context, on the other hand, was not required in this scenario, but it could have been used to describe the morning situation, in so far as it affected some other situations.

User Context was the most relevant contextual information used by this scenario, since it was heavily involved with the user's morning. The user's *Preferences* were instantiated to describe the lighting settings when the user wakes up. In addition, the user has *Activities*, which are used to calculate how much time it takes for the user to actually leave his/her home after waking up, which in this scenario was a predefined time value. In a real scenario, this can be easily picked up by a context monitor that notices when the user leaves the home space, or when the NFC (Near Field Communication) tag is "touched", when physically leaving the home.

The context ontology was used at the development time to add the necessary functionality for both the personal and home space agents. The personal agent communicates with both the spaces, while the home space agent is isolated into the home space. The home space agent only utilizes the home space, so that when security is added into the picture, there's only one space to take care of. All of the relevant devices are expected to have access rights to the home space, so they can add the information which is needed by the home reasoning agent.

We managed to switch on the lighting at the right time, according to the preferences set by the person in the simulated smart home. The only difference to a real situation was that the lighting was simulated with a visualization tool. All of the relevant parts for validating our ontology were done as they would be done in a real situation. That is, the home reasoning agent used our context ontology to find out the person's preferences and ease the morning wake-up as he/she desires, by adjusting the lighting.

In this case, we did not utilize the rules described in the *Digital* Context, besides instantiating a rule, the description of which illuminated what has to be done. For example, adjust the lighting according to the user's preferences at the time that the user is woken up. In the future, we will study how to make the rules updateable via the SIB, so that hard coding these situations will no longer be necessary, as described in [14].

5   Discussions

The core part of SOUPA, one of the ontologies mentioned in the Introduction, is the most similar to our context ontology (CO). The SOUPA also has an extension part for, e.g., supporting specific types of pervasive application domains. Both the CO and the SOUPA core utilize existing ontologies for describing the person and properties needed for pervasive and ubiquitous applications. Our context ontology does not include security concepts for our ontology, like the SOUPA core does. The reason is that we have described security concepts in a separate ontology, Information Security Measurement Ontology (ISMO) [20]. However, we have kept the need for security and privacy in mind by adding the concepts for the role of person, output values which can be, e.g., values from security measurement. We had beliefs, desires and intensions with agents in our initial conceptual context ontology [13] as it is in the SOUPA core. However, our context ontology does not have those for agents anymore, because we decided to use rules for describing the situations that can be desired and the intended behavior for the smart space.

One important thing in the context is the history of it. Our ontology includes a *Historical* Context concept, which can be used to store the whole context if needed. However, since we use the SOFIA SIB, we can directly use our ontology to store old events. For example, one can subscribe to listen to every new *LocationEvent* and receive a notification of every new event that is produced. This can be accomplished by, e.g., adding a new *Event* every time that an *Active Object* has produced one. We can either have only one event at a time, or we can have multiple ones, since the object property is *producesEvent*. Also, the *Contexts* and *Events* have a *Time* property, which can be used to differentiate old and new Events.

In addition, the introduced context ontology is expandable with domain specific parts. The domain specific part is, e.g., the ontology used by the lighting and other smart objects that are controlled via the smart environment. Hence, with the context ontology, we managed to set the desired lighting for the person in his/her smart home.

6   Conclusions and Future Work

In this paper, we introduced the novel and enhanced context ontology that supports building situation-aware applications. Our context ontology for smart spaces, CO4SS, highlights the context through the six context dimensions: physical context, digital context, situational context, user context, historical context, and social context. We used our context ontology in the validation scenario and managed to monitor and reason the necessary information concerning the user in order to wake him up at the right time.

It has been challenging to create the context ontology that is suitable for the heterogeneous smart spaces. Due to the challenges, no results relating to the context ontologies have been recently published. Thus, our goal has been to reach relevant context ontology for smart spaces.

In the future, we will i) concentrate on validating the social and historical parts of our CO4SS ontology, and ii) study how to make the rules updateable via the SIB.

Acknowledgements. This work has been funded by Tekes, VTT, and the European Commission, in the framework of the ARTEMIS JU SP3 SOFIA project.

References

1. Strang, T., Linnhoff-Popien, C., Frank, K.: CoOL: A Context Ontology Language to Enable Contextual Interoperability. In: Stefani, J.-B., Demeure, I., Zhang, J. (eds.) DAIS 2003. LNCS, vol. 2893, pp. 236–247. Springer, Heidelberg (2003)
2. Chen, H., Finin, T., Joshi, A.: An ontology for context-aware pervasive computing environments. Knowledge and Engineering Review, Special Issue on Ontologies for Distributed Systems 18(3), 197–207 (2003)
3. Gu, T., Wang, X., Pung, H.K., Zhang, H.K.: An ontology-based context model in intelligent environments. In: CNDS 2004: The Society for Modeling and Simulation International (SCS), USA, pp. 270–275 (2004)
4. Strimpakou, M., Roussaki, I., Pils, C., Anagnostou, M.: COMPACT: Middleware for context representation and management in pervasive computing environments. International Journal of Pervasive Computing and Communications (JPCC) 2(3), 229–246 (2006)
5. Chen, H., Finin, T., Joshi, A.: The SOUPA ontology for pervasive computing. Whitestein Series in Software Agent Technologies, pp. 233–258. Springer, Heidelberg (2005)
6. Kantrovitch, J., Niemelä, E.: Service Description Ontologies. In: Khosrow-Pour, M. (ed.) Encyclopedia of Information Science and Technology, 2nd edn., vol. VII, R-S, pp. 3445–3451. Published under the imprint Information Science Reference (formerly Idea Group Reference) (2008)
7. Bettini, C., Brdiczka, O., Henricksen, K., Indulska, J., Nicklas, D., Ranganathan, A., Riboni, D.: A survey of context modelling and reasoning techniques. Pervasive and Mobile Computing 6(2), 161–180 (2010)
8. Indulska, J., Nicklas, D.: Introduction to the special issue on context modelling, reasoning and management. Pervasive and Mobile Computing 6(2), 159–160 (2010)
9. Web Ontology Language, http://www.w3.org/TR/owl-features/
10. Soylu, A., De Causmaecker, P., Desmet, P.: Context and Adaptivity in Pervasive Computing Environments: Links with Software Engineering and Ontological Engineering. J. of Software 4(9), 992–1013 (2009)
11. Dey, A. K., Abowd, G. D.: Towards a better understanding of context and context-awareness. Technical Report GIT-GVU-99-22, Georgia Institute of Technology, College of Computing (1999)
12. Toninelli, A., Pantsar-Syväniemi, S., Bellavista, P., Ovaska, E.: Supporting Context Awareness in Smart Environments: a Scalable Approach to Information Interoperability. In: M-MPAC 2010, session: short papers, Article No: 5. IFIP, USENIX. ACM (2009)
13. Pantsar-Syväniemi, S., Simula, K., Ovaska, E.: Context-awareness in Smart Spaces. In: SISS 2010, pp. 1023–1028. IEEE Press, New York (2010)
14. Pantsar-Syväniemi, S., Kuusijärvi, J., Ovaska, E.: Context-Awareness Micro-Architecture for Smart Spaces. In: Riekki, J., Ylianttila, M., Guo, M. (eds.) GPC 2011. LNCS, vol. 6646, pp. 148–157. Springer, Heidelberg (2011)
15. SOFIA IOP, http://www.sofia-project.eu/
16. Resource Description Framework, http://www.w3.org/RDF/
17. Suomalainen, J., Hyttinen, P., Tarvainen, P.: Secure Information Sharing between Heterogeneous Embedded Devices. In: MeSSa 2010, pp. 205–212. ACM Press (2010)
18. Pantsar-Syväniemi, S., Ovaska, E., Ferrari, S., Salmon Cinotti, T., Zamagni, G., Roffia, L., Mattarozzi, S., Nannini, V.: Case Study: Context-aware Supervision of a Smart Maintenance Process. In: SISS 2011, pp. 309–314. IEEE Computer Society (2011)
19. FOAF Vocabulary Specification 0.98, http://xmlns.com/foaf/spec/
20. Evesti, A., Savola, R., Ovaska, E., Kuusijärvi, J.: Design, Instantiation, and Usage of Information Security Measuring Ontology. In: MOPAS 2011, pp. 1–9 (2011)

A Model for Using Machine Learning in Smart Environments

Sakari Stenudd

VTT Technical Research Centre of Finland,
P.O. Box 1100, FIN-90571 Oulu, Finland
Sakari.Stenudd@vtt.fi

Abstract. This work presents a model for using machine learning in the adaptive control of smart environments. The model is based on an investigation of the existing works regarding smart environments and an analysis of the machine learning uses within them. Four different categories of machine learning in smart environments were identified: *prediction, recognition, detection* and *optimisation*. These categories can be deployed to different phases of a self-adaptive application utilising the adaptation loop structure. The use of machine learning in one phase of the adaptation loop was demonstrated by carrying out an experiment utilising neural networks in the prediction of latencies.

Keywords: control loop, adaptive systems, self-adaptive software, prediction.

1 Introduction

There is a number of projects aiming to create smart environments (SEs) [17,21,9], many of which utilise machine learning in some form to improve the operation of the environment [3]. Using machine learning helps in achieving adaptiveness, which in turn helps to reduce the costs of handling the complexity of software systems and in handling unexpected and changed conditions [19].

This paper proposes a model that can be used to categorize uses of machine learning in SEs. Before that, in this section some machine learning terms and SE projects are shortly presented. Based on these, a generic model of using machine learning in SEs is presented in Section 2. The use of the model is demonstrated with an experiment in Section 3, and the results of this work are discussed and compared to other work in Section 4. Finally, Section 5 concludes this paper.

1.1 Machine Learning

This subsection introduces some important terms of machine learning. A machine is said to *learn* if its performance at some defined task or tasks improves with experience [16]. The concept of machine learning can be divided into three subcategories [7]: (1) In *supervised learning* the learning agent has a set of labelled training examples from which it has to generalise a representation; (2) In

M. Rautiainen et al. (Eds.): GPC 2011 Workshops, LNCS 7096, pp. 24–33, 2012.

unsupervised learning no information about the correct output is given; (3) In *reinforcement learning* no desired output is given but the agent receives a reward for every action and it must try to maximise the rewards. Two common problem types for machine learning are *classification* and *regression* problems. In classification problems there is a discrete set of possible outputs and in regression problems the output takes continuous values [16].

There are many data representation formats available for learning [16]: common examples for supervised learning are artificial neural networks, decision trees, rule sets and statistical models, such as hidden Markov models and Bayesian representations (for example naive Bayes). There are also different algorithms which can be used to train the representation model, for example, neural networks can be trained using backpropagation and genetic algorithms can be applied to many models [16]. In data mining, the goal is to find useful information from large sets of data. For this, unsupervised learning techniques are commonly used [2]. In anomaly detection, the goal is to create a model of normal behaviour and detect the deviations from it [18].

1.2   Smart Environment Projects

In smart environments, devices embedded into the environment aim to improve the user experience [4]. Examples of prominent smart environment projects that use machine learning (ML) in some way are ACHE [17], MavHome [21], iDorm [9] and PlaceLab [12]. Their uses of ML are presented below.

In ACHE (Adaptive Control of Home Environments) [17], there are three adaptive component types that use machine learning: device regulators, set-point generators and predictors.

The MavHome (Managing an Intelligent Versatile Home) system [21] uses several machine learning methods in the three phases of its operation. Activity patterns are detected from the observed data using data mining and a prediction algorithm is trained. In addition, an episode membership algorithm, which calculates the probability of a set of observations belonging to a certain episode, is trained using the observation data and activity patterns. For making decisions, a hierarchical hidden Markov model-based model of the environment is created. There is also work done aiming to add anomaly detection capabilities to MavHome [13].

The Essex intelligent Dormitory (iDorm) [9] is a test-bed for ambient intelligence and ubiquitous computing experiments. It learns rules from the behaviour of the user. The learning is based on negative reinforcement and occurs whenever the user expresses dissatisfaction by changing the actions that the embedded agent has carried out.

The PlaceLab [12] is a residential building equipped with a large number of sensors. There has been work mainly on developing activity recognition algorithms which are trained and tested using datasets gathered from the PlaceLab [15].

2   Model

Based on the machine learning uses in existing projects [17,21,13,9,12,15] six machine learning problem types are recognised: (1) event prediction, (2) activity-pattern identification, (3) activity recognition, (4) anomaly detection, (5) device control, and (6) decision making. These can be further divided into four categories. Event prediction belongs to *prediction* problems in which the goal is to create a model that can be used to decide on the most probable subsequent event. Activity recognition is categorised as a *recognition* problem, and its goal is to classify the observed actions to some pre-defined activity. Activity-pattern identification and anomaly detection are *detection* problems in which the goal is to detect frequent patterns occurring in the input data. The last category is *optimisation* problems which contains device control and decision-making problems. In these problems the goal is to find a policy that is optimal in the current situation. The following subsections discuss these problems.

2.1   Detection

Detection problems are typically solved using data-mining algorithms. They divide the training instances into classes according to algorithm-specific criteria. Use of detection algorithms can reduce the amount of work that would be done in labelling training examples for recognition algorithms. However, since the machine does not really know the semantics of the detected situations it may be more challenging to make conclusions based on these situations. For example predefined, rule-based reasoners cannot be used without mapping the detected situations to actual labels.

Anomaly detection is a special case of situation detection when the events are divided into two classes: normal and anomalous. Anomaly detection algorithms are able to detect anomalies even when they occur for the first time.

2.2   Recognition

In this work, recognition problems are classification problems that are handled with supervised learning techniques. The most straightforward way to utilise recognition algorithms in SEs is to train the agent before deploying it to the environment. Online training in the SE may be difficult because agent training requires labelled training examples and they are usually not available at runtime. However, in some cases it may be possible to deduce if the output is right or wrong and thus improve the operation accordingly using, for example, reinforcement learning techniques.

2.3   Prediction

Common to all prediction problems is that their goal is to predict what is going to happen in the near future. The inputs for the predictors can be direct sensor readings or pre-processed information. Prediction problems can be classification or regression problems. An example of classification problems is event prediction, where the goal is to predict the most probable event or subsequent activity, while latency prediction is a regression problem in which the output – the latency value – takes on continuous values.

When prediction agents are used in a SE, online training may be a good approach. For example, a latency predictor can measure the actual latency it was predicting, compare it to the predicted value and improve its future predictions using the actual value as a training example. This requires that the information used in prediction can be coupled with the correct prediction output.

2.4 Optimisation

Problems in which there is the possibility of gaining a reward from the SE and where the goal is to maximise the reward exist within the optimisation category. It is possible to use reinforcement learning for these problems. Some optimisation problems can be handled as prediction problems so that the rewards for different actions are predicted and the action with the highest reward would be chosen. However, the goal of optimisation problems is to find a policy that maximises long-term performance, not just selecting the best next action. Therefore an amount of experimenting with different actions may be advantageous.

Decision making is a good example of an optimisation problem. It requires taking into account many different variables and solving trade-offs between the benefits of different areas of the SE. Another example, device control, may not be present in every SE. It is needed when the devices are given high-level commands and they need to be changed to low-level actuator controls. This may require some experimentation in order to find the optimal way to control the actuators.

2.5 Interaction of Machine Learning Uses

A loop structure is common in adaptive systems. For example the MAPE-K (Monitor, Analyse, Plan, Execute, Knowledge) loop known from the area of autonomic computing [14] is an example of this. Salehie and Tahvildari call the loop the 'adaptation loop' and name the phases as monitoring, detecting, deciding and acting processes [19]. Their work concerns *self-adaptive software* which is a sub-concept of autonomic computing [19]. In this work, the adaptation loop is applied to smart environments.

As can be seen in Figure 1, different machine learning categories identified in this work correspond to different phases of the adaptation loop. The figure shows the adaptation loop [19] with most suitable machine learning categories named for each process. The ML categories are given in parentheses after the process name. Note that the detecting process should not be confused to the detection category: the names are given from different points of view.

Although inspired by autonomic computing, the realisation of this adaptation loop in smart environments will be quite different. In SEs, there are typically a large number of agents, each of which perform a single task and thus the individual agents are very loosely coupled. Therefore, every phase in the loop can

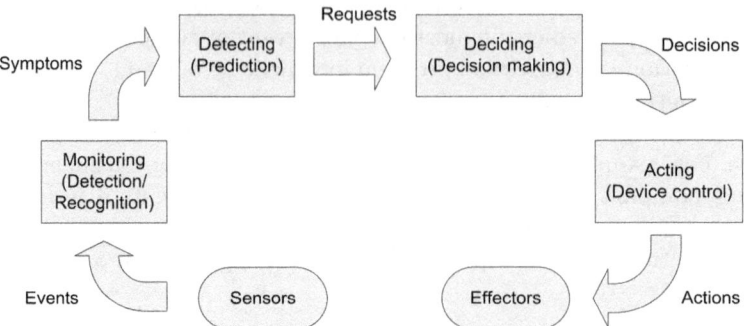

Fig. 1. A model for using machine learning in a smart environment

be implemented in a separate SE agent, and the outputs of agents serve as inputs to other agents. Moreover, actions of some agents or even intermediate results of the loop can serve as "sensor events" to some other agents, thus creating a hierarchical loop structure. Consequently, the actual realisation of the loop may seem a lot more complex than the model in Figure 1.

3 Experiment

In this experiment the goal is to try to improve latency prediction results in a SE using machine learning. The experiment is done in an IOP (Inter-operability Platform) environment [20], in which there are two kinds of software nodes: SIBs (Semantic Information Brokers) and KPs (Knowledge Processors) which communicate using SSAP (Smart Space Access Protocol) operations (see Figure 2). In the IOP, KPs publish and consume information in SIB and thus the SIB acts as a central server through which the information flows. It is obvious that a poorly performing SIB can be a bottleneck in the system. Therefore, the latency of operations made to SIB is chosen to be predicted.

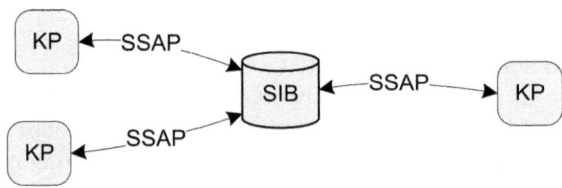

Fig. 2. An information-level view of the IOP

In the adaptation loop of Figure 1, the implemented software module belongs to the detecting process and it helps in determining when adaptation actions should be executed. The measured latencies come from a simple monitoring agent, and based on the predicted latencies, the deciding process could initiate possible adaptation actions before the performance level drops too low due to the load of the SIB.

3.1   Implementation

Two separate agents (KPs) were implemented for the experiment. The first KP, RandomKP, generates load to the SIB. In fact, RandomKP generates many KP instances that connect to the SIB but they are all implemented in one process. It also updates into the SIB the information about (1) the number of joined KPs, (2) the number of triples inserted, and (3) the number of subscriptions made. Thus, RandomKP acts as a monitoring agent in the adaptation loop. The other KP, PredictorKP, tries to predict the amount of time it takes for the SIB to process a query and compares it to the actual time. Both KPs were implemented using C++ language and the Qt toolbox. The SIB used was a non-public Python implementation.

RandomKP provides a user interface (UI) that allows the user control the load generated to the SIB. Using it, it is possible to adjust the rates of generating new KPs and different SSAP operations. The rates can also be given randomly for every generated KP. The different operations that KPs make are query, insert, remove, subscribe and unsubscribe. In the main loop of RandomKP, which runs in its own thread, makes a maximum of one of these operations according to the probabilities given by the user and waits for 1–5 seconds. If the operation affects the number of KPs, triples or subscriptions, the value is updated into the SIB.

PredictorKP is used to train different latency predictors online while making measurements. It makes queries to the SIB in ten seconds intervals and measures the times it takes to receive responses. The predictors are used to predict the latency using the three parameters (numbers of KPs, triples and subscriptions). The predictions are written to a log file and the predictors are trained using the actual latency measurements. PredictorKP provides also a UI to watch the predictions of different predictors.

In this experiment three predictors were implemented: LinearPredictor, Average10Predictor and FFNetPredictor. LinearPredictor and Average10Predictor are very simple predictors and they are used as a reference for testing the neural network implementation FFNetPredictor. LinearPredictor uses the linear function $p_{t+1} = (1-w)p_t + wm$ in which p_t is the prediction at iteration t, m is the latest measured value and w is its weight. The weight decreases from 1 to 0.1 so the later measurements have a greater impact on the prediction. It can be expected to adapt quite slowly to changes in the latencies. Average10Predictor returns the arithmetic average value of ten previous measured latency values as a prediction: $p_t = \frac{1}{10}\sum_{i=1}^{10} m_{t-i}$. Compared to LinearPredictor, this one should react a bit more rapidly to changes in measurements because it only uses ten previous measurements while all measured latencies affect the prediction of LinearPredictor. These predictors do not use the KP, triple and subscription amounts to create the prediction.

FFNetPredictor uses a feed-forward artificial neural network implementation of the Shark machine learning library [10] to create the prediction. The network has three input units, three hidden units and one output which is the latency estimate. The hidden units are sigmoid units, but because they produce results between 0 and 1, the use of them in duration evaluation would require scaling. Therefore the output unit is a linear unit in which the output is a weighted sum of the inputs. Thus the output can be directly used as a duration estimate. The learning algorithm used in the experiment was IRPropPlus [11] which is an improved version of the basic backpropagation training algorithm. The network was trained continuously after each measurement. Thirty previous measurements were saved and used in training. The training algorithm made each time fifty iterations with the thirty training inputs and outputs.

3.2   Evaluation

The applicability of machine learning algorithms used in the experiment was evaluated using the KPs described in the previous section. This section describes one such test run. The Python SIB was run on a Dell Latitude D410 laptop and RandomKP and PredictorKP applications were run on a Dell Latitude D830 laptop. Both machines were in the same local network. The applications were run for about ten minutes and in that time the MeasurerKP made a total of 59 measurements. The three predictors described in the previous section were used to estimate the latency of each query and then the measurement was used to train them. The parameter values of the different measurements are shown in Figure 3a and the measured and estimated latencies are shown in Figure 3b.

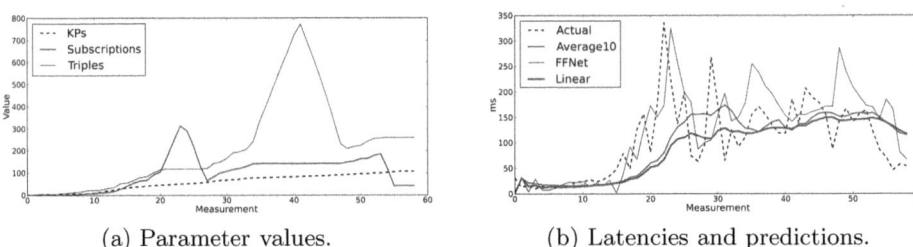

(a) Parameter values.   (b) Latencies and predictions.

Fig. 3. The parameter values, measured latencies and latency estimates of the test run

As can be deduced from the figures, random probabilities for RandomKP instances were used for approximately the first 200 seconds (20 measurements). In this phase, all the used predictors seem to perform quite equally.

When the probability, and consequently the number, of subscriptions is increased, the measured latency also increases dramatically. As expected, the reference predictors do not react very quickly but the FFNetPredictor adapts much better to this change. However, the zigzag curve seen in the figure is very characteristic to the measured latencies and there seems to be no correspondence between this and the used parameter values. Therefore FFNetPredictor is often unable to predict the latencies and seems to be a bit 'late'.

Later when the amount of inserted triples makes a brief peak it can be seen that the change (at least a change of this magnitude) does not substantially affect the latency. However, the FFNetPredictor also makes a short peak when the amount of triples begins to increase. It shows that the predictor had made a false generalisation that the triple amount would affect the latency more but it was able to correct this erroneous assumption.

4   Discussion

The experiment indicates that the use of machine learning techniques can help in predicting latencies, even though there are many possible ways to improve the operation of the learning agent. A more reliable prediction helps in detecting when an adaptation action is needed to ensure that the operation quality of the smart environment remains high.

The main contribution of this work is the model for using machine learning in a smart environment to achieve adaptive control which was presented in Section 2. Although the model was only evaluated using the IOP, the model itself is more generic and it would also work well with other kinds of inter-operability solutions. The benefit of the model comes from the fact that it makes it easier to understand the need and usage of machine learning in SEs. Also, by separating different phases of an adaptation loop into different agents the SE becomes more maintainable, extensible and reusable.

There is still much work to be done in both the areas of machine learning and smart environments. Smart environments can benefit from advances in machine learning and they offer a good application domain in which to develop new learning techniques.

The machine learning model described in Section 2 needs still more validation. In the future, a real smart environment control loop with real physical sensors and actuators using different learning solutions should be created in order to validate the whole model.

4.1   Related Research

There has been other work done regarding the use of machine learning or a sub-concept of it in smart environments. In the MavHome environment machine learning techniques have been in use for quite a long time. Already in 2002, Das et al. [6] described how prediction algorithms were used in MavHome. Their work concentrates on creating a well-working smart home architecture and therefore they only describe the things that are of interest in the MavHome domain. In 2005, Das and Cook [5] also described the need for reinforcement learning in decision making in smart homes. In this work the use of machine learning is presented in a more general form.

In their survey, Aztiria et al. [1] also deal with the use of machine learning in smart environments. They illustrate the SE systems as a three-phase process with sensing, reasoning and acting phases. The reasoning phase consists of activity recognition, learning and decision making phases and contains also knowledge needed in the decision making. This process has many similar characteristics to the model presented in this paper and is also based on a survey of existing work. The greatest difference is in that they see the SE more as a system with a fixed process, and in our work the SE is thought to be more complex and have many such hierarchical processes.

Fernandez-Montes et al. [8] also propose a loop structure for smart environments. Their loop consists of three phases: perception, reasoning and acting. These main tasks are further divided into different sub-tasks. In their architecture, all the learning capabilities are included in the reasoning phase in which many different learning tasks are contained in a learning agent. Thus, in their model, extending the capabilities of the SE would always need modification of the monolithic learning agent.

5   Conclusions

This paper described the general uses of machine learning techniques in some of the existing smart environment projects. Based on these works, there were four different categories of machine learning uses found: (1) detection, (2) recognition, (3) prediction, and (4) optimisation.

A model based on a loop structure for autonomically managing devices in the smart environment using machine learning was proposed. The loop consists of the aforementioned categories combined to a generic adaptation loop.

To demonstrate the use of the resulting model, a test experiment was carried out and classified according to the model. It was a latency predictor, which could be positioned to the detecting process of the presented adaptation loop. It was able to predict the latencies better than simpler reference predictors in certain situations.

Acknowledgements. The work presented in this paper was carried out as a part of the TIVIT/DIEM project. I would like to thank Anu Purhonen for her helpful comments during this work.

References

1. Aztiria, A., Izaguirre, A., Augusto, J.C.: Learning patterns in ambient intelligence environments: a survey. Artificial Intelligence Review 34(1), 35–51 (2010)
2. Berkhin, P.: A survey of clustering data mining techniques. In: Grouping Multidimensional Data, pp. 25–71. Springer, Heidelberg (2006)
3. Cook, D.J., Das, S.K.: Smart Environments: Technologies, Protocols, and Applications. John Wiley, Hoboken (2005)
4. Cook, D.J., Das, S.K.: How smart are our environments? an updated look at the state of the art. Pervasive and Mobile Computing 3(2), 53–73 (2007)

5. Das, S.K., Cook, D.J.: Designing Smart Environments: A Paradigm Based on Learning and Prediction. In: Pal, S.K., Bandyopadhyay, S., Biswas, S. (eds.) PReMI 2005. LNCS, vol. 3776, pp. 80–90. Springer, Heidelberg (2005)
6. Das, S.K., Cook, D.J., Battacharya, A., Heierman III, E.O., Lin, T.Y.: The role of prediction algorithms in the mavhome smart home architecture. IEEE Wireless Communications 9(6), 77–84 (2002)
7. Duda, R.O., Hart, P.E., Stork, D.G.: Pattern Classification, 2nd edn. John Wiley, New York (2001)
8. Fernandez-Montes, A., Ortega, J.A., Alvarez, J.A., Gonzalez-Abril, L.: Smart environment software reference architecture. In: Fifth International Joint Conference on INC, IMS and IDC, NCM 2009, August 25-27, pp. 397–403 (2009)
9. Hagras, H., Callaghan, V., Colley, M., Clarke, G., Pounds-Cornish, A., Duman, H.: Creating an ambient-intelligence environment using embedded agents. IEEE Intelligent Systems 19(6), 12–20 (2004)
10. Igel, C., Glasmachers, T., Heidrich-Meisner, V.: Shark. Journal of Machine Learning Research 9, 993–996 (2008)
11. Igel, C., Hüsken, M.: Empirical evaluation of the improved Rprop learning algorithms. Neurocomputing 50(1), 105–124 (2003)
12. Intille, S.S., Larson, K., Tapia, E.M., Beaudin, J.S., Kaushik, P., Nawyn, J., Rockinson, R.: Using a Live-in Laboratory for Ubiquitous Computing Research. In: Fishkin, K.P., Schiele, B., Nixon, P., Quigley, A. (eds.) PERVASIVE 2006. LNCS, vol. 3968, pp. 349–365. Springer, Heidelberg (2006)
13. Jakkula, V.R., Crandall, A.S., Cook, D.J.: Enhancing anomaly detection using temporal pattern discovery. In: Advanced Intelligent Environments, pp. 175–194. Springer, US (2009)
14. Kephart, J.O., Chess, D.M.: The vision of autonomic computing. IEEE Computer 36(1), 41–50 (2003)
15. Logan, B., Healey, J., Philipose, M., Tapia, E.M., Intille, S.S.: A Long-Term Evaluation of Sensing Modalities for Activity Recognition. In: Krumm, J., Abowd, G.D., Seneviratne, A., Strang, T. (eds.) UbiComp 2007. LNCS, vol. 4717, pp. 483–500. Springer, Heidelberg (2007)
16. Mitchell, T.M.: Machine learning. McGraw-Hill, New York (1997)
17. Mozer, M.C.: The neural network house: An environment that adapts to its inhabitants. In: Proc. AAAI Spring Symposium on Intelligent Environments (1998)
18. Patcha, A., Park, J.M.: An overview of anomaly detection techniques: Existing solutions and latest technological trends. Computer Networks 51(12), 3448–3470 (2007)
19. Salehie, M., Tahvildari, L.: Self-adaptive software: Landscape and research challenges. ACM Trans. Auton. Adapt. Syst. 4, 14:1–14:42 (2009)
20. Toninelli, A., Pantsar-Syväniemi, S., Bellavista, P., Ovaska, E.: Supporting context awareness in smart environments: a scalable approach to information interoperability. In: Proceedings of the International Workshop on Middleware for Pervasive Mobile and Embedded Computing, pp. 1–4. ACM (2009)
21. Youngblood, G.M., Cook, D.J., Holder, L.B.: Managing adaptive versatile environments. Pervasive and Mobile Computing 1(4), 373–403 (2005)

Flexible Security Deployment in Smart Spaces

Jani Suomalainen

VTT Technical Research Centre of Finland
Espoo, Finland
Jani.Suomalainen@vtt.fi

Abstract. Smart spaces, which utilize publish and subscribe architectures as well as semantic information, promise to ease cooperation of heterogeneous devices. To make smart spaces feasible for open multi-user environments we must provide easy-to-use security solutions. In this paper, we focus on security deployment issues, particularly to credential establishment and configuration of access control. The paper concentrates on challenges caused by heterogeneity of devices as well as dynamic nature of users, authorities, and security policies. To address these issues, the paper describes how credentials can be deployed in Smart Space architecture and how access control policies can be generated using available semantic information. Finally, the paper describes security implementations for a Semantic Information Broker and for Device Interconnect Protocol.

Keywords: smart space, security establishment, credentials, access control, reasoning.

1   Introduction

The amount of different networked devices and availability of communication mechanisms is rapidly increasing. This has made possible to develop new kinds of applications, where devices cooperate and utilize information available in the surrounding physical environment. To ease this cooperation, gateways and semantic interoperability solutions have been introduced and utilized, e.g. in smart spaces [1].

Smart spaces consist of two kinds of dynamic architectural components. Knowledge Processors (KP) generate, publish, subscribe, modify and consume information. Semantic Information Brokers (SIB) store and forward information. Smart spaces may be build on top of different connectivity mechanisms, such as TCP/IP or Bluetooth, or middleware approaches such Device Interconnect Protocol [2]. Semantic interoperability solutions [3] include eXtensible Markup Language (XML) for data encoding and Resource Description Framework (RDF) for knowledge representation. To ease information sharing, ontology description languages such as RDF Schema, and Web Ontology Language are used to define semantic meaning for data, i.e. to define the concepts, properties, and their relations, for different domains. With different reasoning rules we can then perform more intelligent actions and derive new information from existing data and semantic knowledge.

M. Rautiainen et al. (Eds.): GPC 2011 Workshops, LNCS 7096, pp. 34–43, 2012.

RDF Information Base Solution (RIBS) is one SIB implementation. In [4] we described our solution for securing communication between RIBS and knowledge processors. The paper described how brokering devices may measure the security level of communication sessions and authorize information access using this information. Further, the paper surveyed some related research. In [5] we described requirements for smart space security and presented a complete implementation of fine-grained access control system for RIBS. In [6] we surveyed technologies for key establishment in personal communication standards.

In this paper, we focus on smart space specific security deployment issues. We contribute by describing how credentials can be distributed and how security policies can be applied easily in smart spaces. Section 2 describes challenges met in heterogeneous and dynamic spaces. In Section 3, we propose credential and security deployment solutions for architecture and policy management. Section 4 presents our security implementation from security deployment point of view. Further, the section will describe examples of models for deriving access control policies from semantic information.

2   Security Deployment Challenges for Smart Space Platforms

This section lists security challenges that developers must consider when designing platforms for smart spaces.

2.1   Credential Management for Heterogeneous Technologies

Major security requirements such as confidentiality, integrity, availability, access control, privacy and non-repudiation are dependent on reliable and secure key establishment and deployment mechanisms. Devices must acquire keys and credentials, which enable them to prove their trustworthiness and authorizations for other peers and verify others trustworthiness. When a smart space supports various security protocols, we need to deliver different kinds of credentials. Also, as smart spaces are heterogeneous it is not likely that single credential deployment model is sufficient. Therefore, we need to consider different scenarios.

Scenario A – Shared Secret for Public Key Certificates. Devices or KPs, with more processing capacity, may establish session keys using certificates and private keys. These certificates can be requested from certifier, which all parties trust. One approach to control that keys are delivered to correct parties is to protect certificate requests and deliveries with pre-shared secret. This is straightforward approach with some usability and security constrains related to delivery and length of the unique secret.

Scenario B – Out of Band Models for Symmetric Credentials and Low Cost Security. Low resource devices may not be able to secure communication with private – public key pairs. One approach is to deliver symmetric network keys using trusted of band channels such as Near Field Communication (NFC) or Universal Serial Bus (USB). Some out-of-band models are bi-directional and some one-directional, which will further complicate the deployment. In smart spaces, trusted brokers may forward device specific keys to other devices. The key exchange may need to be controlled by security authorities and forwarding needs to be controlled by users. Further, when forwarding credentials to other devices, we need to consider trust issues. However, devices without direct security relationships may not know how trustworthy mechanisms have been used when keys where initially deployed to the broker.

Scenario C – End-User Specific Secrets for Access from Shared Devices. End-users may use shared or borrowed devices to access data. In these cases we cannot assume availability of existing credentials in devices. It should be possible for users to use e.g. passwords, biometrics or security tokens to access data.

2.2   Dynamic Devices, Shared Brokers and Multiple Authorities

Smart spaces are dynamic. Users, devices and brokers may join and leave at any time. Therefore, spaces should not assume availability of any component. Further, in some smart spaces there may be multiple distrusting authorities. These authorities may control same SIBs and want to ensure that only those devices, which are certified by them, can access shared information. For example, buildings may have devices, which are shared by several families, and malls may have devices used to serve different shops. Therefore, smart space platforms should provide solutions for adding new authorities. Since also authorities may emerge any time, these mechanisms should be dynamic and preferably not involve actions from SIB provider. Mechanisms should also be provided to enable users to determine trustworthiness of authorities.

2.3   Dynamic Permission Assignment

Credential deployment and permission assignment mechanism must be self-managing as devices or users may join or leave smart spaces at any time. Since we want new users to be able to access existing data, they must be provided sufficient credentials at any time. This is challenging when the security authority, who certifies users, is not joined to smart space at the time. Also, even if the authority would be available it would not be feasible that the authority would have to manually change permissions for every piece of information within the broker.

When an unknown user joins a smart space, only minimal permissions can be given at default. If a trusted party can verify users trustworthiness or if user can verify its own trustworthiness (e.g. via membership to a trusted group), more permissions can be given. These permissions can then be enforced by checking whether a user trying to access information has required qualifications (e.g. is a member of particular group). However, this approach is problematic due to difficulty of permission revocation (e.g. instead of revocating a permission from a member we would have to revocate permissions from the whole group). Therefore, a better approach would be to automatically set which pieces of information in the broker are accessible for this particular user.

3   Security Deployment Solutions for Smart Spaces

This section proposes generic solutions for deploying security to smart spaces. Particularly, the section describes how new users, devices and security authorities are added and security relationships established. Then, the section describes how access control policies can be automatically generated so that addition of new devices or users does require additional configuration.

3.1   Credential Deployment Architecture

The proposed credential deployment architecture utilizes RDF information sharing mechanisms available in the smart spaces. The architecture consist of three components: KPs (or device or end-user, wishing to access smart space), SIBs (relaying credential information) and security authorities (SAs). The architecture is logical. SIB and SA may locate in the same physical device. Basic KP functionality (client-side communication with SIB) is extended with software enabling it to communicate directly with SA devices. An example of architecture with multiple authorities is illustrated in Fig. 1.

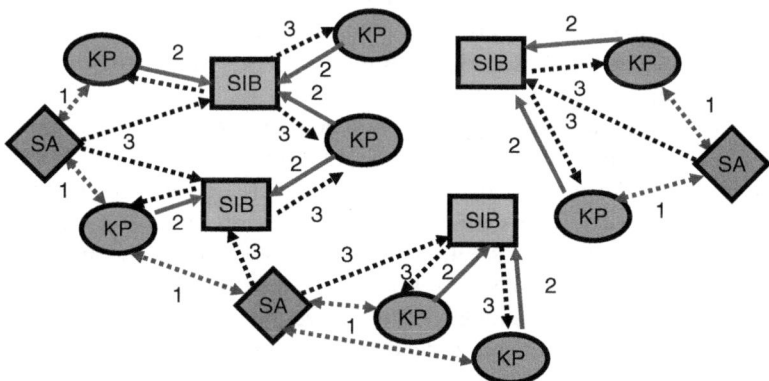

Fig. 1. Smart space architecture example with brokers (SIB), knowledge processors (KPs) and multiple security authoritys (SAs). Blue arrow (1) illustrates key establishment, red arrow (2) KP registration and black arrows (3) credential delivery.

The credential deployment has the following main steps:
1   SA and KP establish a shared secret. SA may also deliver credentials (e.g. X509 root certificates) which enable KP to verify SIBs trustworthiness. Shared secret can be established using various mechanisms (see [6] for some standardized examples). Some end-user contribution is required.
2   KP registers itself to SIB
2.1 KP creates requests for each technology specific credential it requires. The request is encrypted with the shared secret and contains identity information. E.g. in case X509 certificates are requested, certificate's name and public key is stored

to SIB. In case of username-password pair, KP stores either the username or the pair. In case of symmetric encryption, only device ID need to be stored.

2.2 KP stores credential request (e.g. certificate requests) to SIB. SIB notifies those SAs, which have subscribed information on new credential requests.

3   SA provides credentials for KP through SIB and sets access control policies

3.1 SA decrypts requests and generates credentials. Information on how shared secret was established as well as optional trust information is stored to credentials (e.g. to X509 certificate's subject name or alternative name fields). SA encrypts credentials with shared secret and stores them to SIB. KP is notified.

3.2 SA modifies KP's information in SIB so that KP gains correct permissions. For instance, KP may be added to particular groups or given particular roles. Permission assignment is based on information, which can be collected in step 1 (e.g. by SA querying end-user what roles are given for KP). User information is made accessible only for the KP and SA.

3.3 KP downloads credentials from SIB and decrypts them

3.4 KP may upload credentials enabling other KPs to interoperate with it directly. These credentials are protected by setting appropriate access control policies.

The advantage of this indirect credential establishment is that SIB can distribute any kind of credentials. Hence, if we have e.g. created security session with Bluetooth, the end-user is not required to perform any more actions in order to use also TLS or wireless local area network security within the same space. Also, KP can get credentials, which enable device to directly contact other devices in smart space. Further, KPs may use this same approach to renew existing credentials. Of course, it is possible to deliver credentials and some permissions, directly at step 1, without the overhead of step 3. However, when SA sets KP's security attributes directly to SIB it can more flexibly control KP's permissions. E.g. by modifying role assignment it can add and revoke some permissions without revoking the whole credential.

The secret established in the step 1 is used for protection against man-in-the-middle attacks. However, the strength of this secret depends on the method that was used to establish it. If possible, the credentials will contain information identifying the credential delivery method. This trust information is later on used when making authorization decisions. For example, if Bluetooth pairing mechanism is consider to be weak, the KP cannot use TLS session to gain access to critical information.

The model provides flexibility as it enables that SA does not need to be available when KP registers to SIB, SIBs do not need to be available when KP and SA make connection, and KP does not have to be available when credentials have been created. Access to SIB is gained when it becomes available and more permissions are gained when also SA joins smart space.

SIBs can enforce policies coming from devices, which have been certified by different SAs, this is needed to keep certification process lighter (as one authority does not need to do all operations), and more secure (as authorities do not need to trust each other). Before the deployment scenario illustrate above is possible, SA and SIB must establish trust relation. In this phase, SA delivers credentials (e.g. X509 root certificates or shared secrets), enabling SIB to verify KPs.

3.2   Run-Time Policy Generation

KPs storing information and SAs authorizing KPs need to control which users in which context can perform which actions to which information pieces. This control is done to the access control matrices, which SIB enforces. Access control matrices can be presented as a cube, which is a large data structure with information pieces in one dimension, users and context rules in one dimension and actions such as read or write in one dimension. Truth values in matrices then indicate whether action is allowed or denied. In larger environments with multiple users and large amount of data, the size of access control matrices may become large. The management of matrices is challenging if every permission must be set explicitly.

To ease this configuration, we propose that security policies are automatically derived from existing data using semantic information on the security relations. For policy generation we need tools, which are able look semantic relations of existing data and then generate new data and which are easy for developers. For instance, reasoning rules, which can be implemented using logic languages, may be used for this purpose. One reasoning solution is the Answer Set Programming (ASP) paradigm [7].

Semantic data, which rules utilize, can be based on models, which already exists in the security field. For instance, we can utilize role based access control [8], where users are assigned roles giving them access to particular assets. Further, we may utilize classifications of security mechanisms based on evaluated security strength (e.g. [6]).

Fig. 2. illustrates how semantic information in ontologies are used to by rules to derive data for access control cube. A simple example could be a user, who has family roles or work assignments. These roles or assignments are related to particular information, which must be available for the user. By scanning existing data rule the solver would notice that there are users with these relations and information whose access is authorized by these relations. The solver can also check that trust grating given for the user fulfils security requirements, which the author of the information has set. Based on this reasoning, the solver can add new entries to access control matrices.

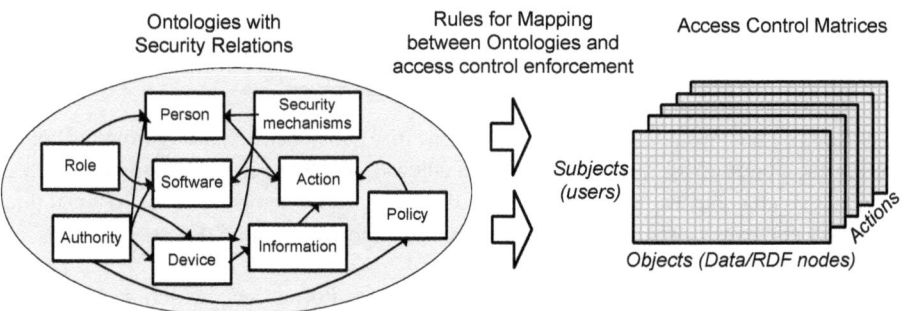

Fig. 2. Mapping security properties from ontologies to the RDF access control matrices. Security relevant semantic data related to user and RDF nodes is derived from ontologies using reasoning rules in order to add entries into access control matrices.

The proposed reasoning can be done at the time when information is accessed. Alternatively, to optimize check times reasoning can be done before hand, particularly, when new users are added (Step 3.2 in Subsection 3.1) or when information related to policies is changed (e.g. a security relations related to information is changed). In the revocation, automatically generated policies must be kept separate from explicitly added policies. This is enabled by adding additional entries to action dimension (e.g. in the matrice levels in of Fig. 2 we have actions 'readAllowed' and 'readAllowedByReasoning').

It is critical that rules work correctly i.e. they provide sufficient coverage and won't act maliciously. Therefore, we can only trust rules coming from trusted sources. One deployment possibility is that SIB provider specifies and deploys supported security rules and ontologies. Alternatively, SAs could deliver and register own security ontologies and rules. SIBs need to advertise, which ontologies and rules they support. KP, which knows that its data is supported by these security rules, does not make any additional access control operations. KP, which does not know that rules cover its data but which handles critical data, must explicitly specify low-level access control policies.

4   Implementation

This section describes our security implementations for a smart space platform. The security has been implemented to several components in RIBS communication software stack and to security KPs as illustrated in Fig. 3.

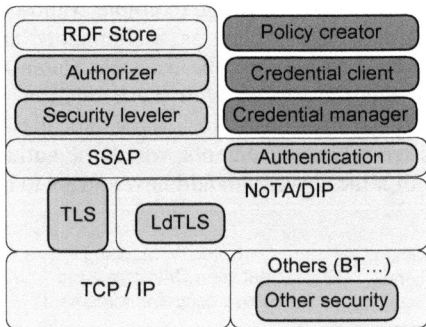

Fig. 3. RIBS communication software stack and security components. Starting from the bottom there are the connectivity alternatives with middleware communication solutions on top of them. Dark green components in the top right illustrate security components for KPs and three components in the opposite left provide access control enforcement for RIBS.

Lowest layer of the figure contains connectivity alternatives, which may be used by Smart Space Access Protocol (SSAP) directly or through Device Interconnect Protocol (DIP). Communication security is achieved with Smart Space Access Protocol / Transmission Layer Security (TLS), Device Interconnect Protocol with TLS (DIP/LdTLS) or with connectivity (such as Bluetooth) specific mechanisms. There is also a complementing end-user authentication solution in the SSAP layer. Security leveler and authorizer components are used to control, which users are allowed to access RDF store. Additionally, we need programs for controlling access control policies and for credential management.

4.1 DIP Security

Device Interconnect Protocol (DIP) [2] is a middleware communication solution, which is a key building block of Network over Terminal Architecture (NoTA). DIP provides consistent socket API for application developers and hides protocol details such as addresses. DIP implementations provide adapters for different transport protocols such as TCP/IP and Bluetooth.

The security has been implemented as a new TLS adapter (named LdTLS) provides a security solution for connection oriented communication. LdTLS uses OpenSSL library's TLS/SSL protocol implementation to encrypt and authenticate TCP/IP communication. The implementation is an extension to LdTCP module. In LdTLS, TCP operations have been replaced with TLS operations. When there are several adapters build to the stack, LdTLS is selected by setting priorities. Deployment of credentials and TLS specific parameters through the DIP stack was enabled by extending the address structure with credentials and by providing socket option call for delivering security information to adapters.

4.2 RIBS Security

Security in RIBS is based on communication security components under the SSAP layer. These components may be either the DIP security solutions or RIBS specific solutions. The RIBS specific TLS solution can use either OpenSSL and GnuTLS libraries. RIBS provides necessary credentials enabling components to authenticate peers and protect communication. When a KP joins RIBS, credentials and information on security parameters (communication protocol, ciphers, credential deployment mechanisms etc.) are passed for the security leveler and authorizer components. The leveler normalizes security parameters so that authorizer may use information from different security components when controlling access to RDF store.

Authorizer makes fine grained access control decisions on the RDF node level. For each node, it is possible to define different security policies, stating e.g. which users are allowed to read data or who is the authority. Additionally, it is possible to set requirements for the security strength level or trustworthiness of the KP or communication session. X509 certificates are used by TLS layer to incorporate information on the identities belonging to the user as well as on the trustworthiness of the user. An authenticated user may have several active identities and states including end user, device, and group (e.g. role) identities as well as security levels. Each identity and state may authorize the user to access particular information. Security policies are stored by any user, who has sufficient permissions to do so. As policies are sent as RDF triplets and stored to subject-predicate-object cube of RIBS, no security specific mechanism for policy delivery or storage is needed. Policies can be set explicitly for each node or they can be implicitly derived using ontologies as described in the following subsection.

4.3 Policy Generation Models

We use the Answer Set Programming (ASP) solver [7] to resolve access control policies from existing data and ontologies. The models have been implemented as lparse programs for smodels [9] solver. This subsection presents few examples on how new policies can be derived.

Fig. 4 illustrates a simple scenario where a rule, presented in one line, is used to find authorized relations. The example data contains few nodes, presenting smart space devices, which are classified to asset domains. Example data contains also few roles, which are given access to domains. The example contains also new a triplet for new user, which is assigned to 'guards' role. Finally, the authorized rule is used to find all authorized user-device pairs. The example assumes that all authorizations have been configured by setting 'canControl. policy relations between roles and asset domains. The example can easily extended to support different ontologies and e.g. hierarchical policy models.

```
% Example RDF data:
belongs (thermostat,climate).        % Node and its domain
belongs (lock,security).             % Node and its domain
canControl (guards, security).       % Role-domain policy
canControl (salespersons, climate).  % Role-domain policy
memberOf (new_guard,guards).         % New user and its role


% Rule for finding authorized relations:
authorized(U,N)  :- memberOf(U,G),belongs(N,D),canControl(G,D).
```

Fig. 4. Example RDF data and a (lparse) logic program for resolving authorizing relations

The example can be extended by considering trust level in authorization. In Fig. 5, we state that security in the credential deployment of a new guard was based on pairing in Bluetooth 2.0 and give this mechanism a security level 2. Then we create main power switch and require that users must be in the level 3. Finally, we add rules which check that the user has sufficient security level. In the example, no 'AuthorizedTrusted' relations are found.

```
belongs (mainPowerSwitch, security).
requiresSecurity (mainPowerSwitch, level3).
credentialsDeployedWith(new_guard, bluetoothv20).
hasSecurityGrade (bluetoothv20, level2).

% New rules:
hasTrustGrade (U, T)  :- credentialsDeployedWith(U,C),
                         hasSecurityGrade(C,T).
isTrusted (U, N)  :- hasTrustGrade(U,T), requiresSecurity(N,T).
authorizedTrusted(U,N)  :-hasAuthorization(U,N), isTrusted(U,N).
```

Fig. 5. RDF data and rule extensions for verifying trust levels required in authorization

5   Conclusions

Strong security mechanisms are difficult to make completely transparent for the end users. However, we can create smart spaces, where fine-grained security configuration is possible with minimal interactions from the end users or security administrators. The key enabler for this security configuration is broker-centric credential deployment architecture. Also, the reasoning and policy generation based on measured and semantic information as well as logic rules seems to be a promising approach, which requires further research in the future. With the help of flexible standards for semantic information, mechanisms for easily providing semantic information, and models for security reasoning, developers may more easily provide solutions which will work securely in any environment.

Acknowledgements. This work was done within EU/ARTEMIS project SOFIA (Smart Objects For Intelligent Applications), which has been funded by Tekes (the Finnish Funding Agency for Technology and Innovation), EU and VTT. Kari Keinänen helped in DIP development and Pasi Hyttinen helped with RIBS and reasoning. Special thanks for Eila Ovaska and the S3E workshop reviewers and participants for valuable feedback.

References

1. Honkola, J., Laine, H., Brown, R., Oliver, I.: Cross-Domain Interoperability: A Case Study. In: Balandin, S., Moltchanov, D., Koucheryavy, Y. (eds.) ruSMART 2009. LNCS, vol. 5764, pp. 22–31. Springer, Heidelberg (2009)
2. NoTAWorld. DIP - Device Interconnect Protocol,
   http://www.notaworld.org/nota/dip
3. World Wide Web Consortium, http://www.w3.org
4. Suomalainen, J., Hyttinen, P., Tarvainen, P.: Secure Information Sharing between Heterogeneous Embedded Devices. In: Proceedings of the Fourth European Conference on Software Architecture: Companion (2010)
5. Suomalainen, J., Hyttinen, P.: Security Solutions for Smart Spaces. To appear in the Proceedings of the Second International Workshop on Semantic Interoperability for Smart Spaces (SISS 2011), Munich, Germany, July 18-22 (2011)
6. Suomalainen, J., Valkonen, J., Asokan, N.: Standards for Security Associations in Personal Networks: A Comparative Analysis. International Journal of Security and Networks 4(1/2), 87–100 (2009)
7. Niemelä, I.: Logic programs with stable model semantics as a constraint programming paradigm. Annals of Mathematics and Artificial Intelligence 25(3), 241–273 (1999)
8. Ferraiolo, D., Kuhn, R.: Role-Based Access Control. In: The 15th National Computer Security Conference (1992)
9. Niemelä, I., Simons, P.: Smodels - An Implementation of the Stable Model and Well-Founded Semantics for Normal LP. In: Fuhrbach, U., Dix, J., Nerode, A. (eds.) LPNMR 1997. LNCS, vol. 1265, pp. 421–430. Springer, Heidelberg (1997)

Using Semantic Transformers to Enable Interoperability between Media Devices in a Ubiquitous Computing Environment

Gerrit Niezen, Bram van der Vlist, Jun Hu, and Loe Feijs

Department of Industrial Design, Technische Universiteit Eindhoven
Den Dolech 2, 5612 AZ Eindhoven, The Netherlands
{g.niezen,b.j.j.v.d.vlist,j.hu,l.m.g.feijs}@tue.nl

Abstract. One of the aims of ubiquitous computing is to enable "serendipitous interoperability"; i.e., to make devices that were not necessarily designed to work together interoperate with one another. It also promises to make technologies disappear, by weaving themselves into the fabric of everyday life until they are indistinguishable from it. In order to reach this goal, self-configuration of the various devices and technologies in ubicomp environments is essential. Whether automated and initiated by context-aware entities, or initiated by users by creating *semantic connections* between devices, the actual configuration of the various components (based on their capabilities) should be performed automatically by the system. In this paper we introduce *semantic transformers* that can be employed to enable interoperability through self-configuration mechanisms.

Keywords: semantic transformers, interoperability, self-configuring systems, Semantic Web, ontology.

1 Introduction

A key goal of ubiquitous computing [13] is "serendipitous interoperability", where devices which were not necessarily designed to work together (e.g. built for different purposes by different manufacturers at different times) should be able to discover each others' functionality and be able to make use of it [2]. Future ubiquitous computing scenarios involve hundreds of devices, appearing and disappearing as their owners carry them from one room or building to another. Therefore, standardizing all the devices and usage scenarios a priori is an unmanageable task.

One possible solution to solving the interoperability problem through self-configuration is being formulated as part of a software platform developed within the SOFIA project[1]. SOFIA (Smart Objects For Intelligent Applications) is a European research project that attempts to make information in the physical

---

[1] http://www.sofia-project.eu/

M. Rautiainen et al. (Eds.): GPC 2011 Workshops, LNCS 7096, pp. 44–53, 2012.
© Springer-Verlag Berlin Heidelberg 2012

world available for smart services — connecting the physical world with the information world. The centre of the software platform developed within SOFIA is a common, semantic-oriented store of information and device capabilities called a Semantic Information Broker (SIB). Various virtual and physical smart objects, termed Knowledge Processors (KPs), interact with one another through the SIB. The goal is that devices will be able to interact on a semantic level, utilizing (potentially different) existing underlying services or service architectures.

Ontologies lend themselves well for describing the characteristics of devices, the means to access such devices, and other technical constraints and requirements that affect incorporating a device into a smart environment [2]. Using an ontology also simplifies the process of integrating different device capability descriptions, as the different entities and relationships in the SIB can be referred to unambiguously. Because communication via the SIB is standardized, integrating cross-vendor implementations is also simplified, and technical incompatibilities can be captured by the ontology.

Next to "serendipitous interoperability", another key goal of ubiquitous computing is to make technologies — as from a user's perspective they are still dealing with technologies — disappear, and weave themselves into the fabric of everyday life until they are indistinguishable from it [13]. To reach this goal, self-configuration of the various devices and technologies in ubicomp environments is essential. Whether automated and initiated by context-aware entities, or initiated by users through establishing *semantic connections* (as introduced in [12,11]) the actual configuration of the various components at a lower level should happen automatically. In this paper we introduce *semantic transformers* that can be employed to enable interoperability between different devices in a ubiquitous computing environment. This is done using self-configuration mechanisms that utilize device capability descriptions to determine how devices may interoperate, either directly or through semantic transformers.

2   Related Work

Various technologies have been developed to discover and describe device capabilities in order to solve the interoperability problem. Universal Plug-and-Play (UPnP) with its device control protocols is one of the more successful solutions[2]. However, it has no task decomposition hierarchy and only allows for the definition of one level of tasks [9].

Current RDF-based schemas for representing information about device capabilities include W3C's CC/PP (Composite Capability/Preference Profiles) and WAP Forum's UAProf (The User Agent Profile) specification. UAProf is used to describe the capabilities of mobile devices, and distinguishes between hardware and software components for devices.

A number of ontologies have been developed for ubiquitous computing environments that may potentially be used to describe device capabilities. Chen et al. [3] defined SOUPA, a context ontology based on OWL (Web Ontology

---

[2] http://upnp.org/sdcps-and-certification/standards/sdcps/

Language), to support ubiquitous agents in their Context Broker Architecture (CoBrA). The ontology supports describing devices on a very basic level (e.g. typical object properties are `bluetoothMAC` or `modelNumber`), but it has no explicit support for modeling more general device capabilities.

Ngo et al. [8] developed the CAMUS ontology in OWL to support context awareness in ubiquitous environments. Their device ontology is based on the FIPA device ontology specification[3], with every `Device` having the properties of `hasHWProfile`, `hasOwner`, `hasService` and `hasProductInfo`. Devices are further classified into `AudioDevice`, `MemoryDevice`, `DisplayDevice`, or `Network-Device`. For audio, the `hasParameter` property has the `AudioParameter` class as range, with subclasses like `ACDCParameter`, `Intensity` and `HarmonicityRatio`. Unfortunately it does not define a notion of completeness, and the ontology is thus not considered generic enough for general use in ubicomp environments.

The SPICE Mobile Ontology[4] allows for the definition of device capabilities in a sub-ontology called Distributed Communication Sphere (DCS) [10]. A distinction is made between device capabilities, modality capabilities and network capabilities. While the ontology provides for a detailed description of the different modality capabilities, e.g. being able to describe force feedback as a `TactileOutputModalityCapability`, there are no subclass assertions made for other device capabilities. Most physical characteristics of the devices are described via their modality capabilities, e.g. a `screenHeight` data property extends the `VisualModalityCapability` with an integer value, and the `audioChannels` data property is also related to an integer value with `Acoustic-ModalityCapability`. The input format of audio content is described via the `AcousticInputModalityCapability` through an `inputFormat` data property to a string value.

It is not clear whether the modality capabilities should be used to describe the actual content that may be exchanged or the user interaction capabilities. As an example, if a device has an `AcousticOutputModalityCapability`, it is not clear whether the device can provide user interaction feedback (e.g. in the form of computer-generated speech or an audible click), or that the device has a speaker.

3   Semantic Connections

As described in the introduction, *semantic connections* were introduced as a means for users to indicate their intentions concerning the information exchange between smart objects in a smart environment. The term semantic connections is used in the context of the SOFIA project to refer to meaningful connections and relationships between entities in a smart environment. We envision these connections as both real "physical" connections (e.g. wired or wireless connections that exist in the real world) and "mental" conceptual connections that seem to be there from a user's perspective. Their context (things they connect)

---

[3] http://www.fipa.org/specs/fipa00091/SI00091E.html
[4] http://ontology.ist-spice.org/

is pivotal for their meaning. The term "semantics" refers to the meaningfulness of the connections. We consider the type of connection, which often has the emphasis now (e.g. WiFi, Bluetooth or USB) not to be the most relevant, but what the connection can do for someone — its functionality — even more.

Semantic connections exist in both the physical and the digital world. They have informative properties, i.e., they are perceivable in the physical world and have sensory qualities that inform users about their uses. The digital counterparts of semantic connections are modeled in an ontology. There may be very direct mappings, e.g. a connection between two real-world entities may be modelled by a `connectedTo` relationship in the ontology. Semantic connections can exist between the following entities: artifacts, smart objects, sensors, UI elements, places, (smart) spaces and persons. Semantic connections have properties like directionality, symmetry, transitivity, reflexiveness and modality.

Crucial to our approach is to make the gap between user goal and action smaller. If we consider streaming music from one device to another, "streaming" now consists of multiple actions that do not necessarily make sense to a user, but are necessary from a technological perspective. In our view, this single high-level goal should have one single high-level action, or at least as few actions as possible. The actual configuration of the devices, i.e., matching device capabilities, transforming content or information to the format that is accepted by the receiving device and negotiating passwords and permissions should happen automatically, based on the user's goals and the constraints of the environment. Our earlier work on mapping the user needs to the actual configurations of the devices uses an heuristic approach at mostly syntactic level [5,6,7]. In this work this is improved by the semantic transformers. In the following two sections we describe how to model device capabilities and relate them to user actions through the use of semantic transformers.

4   Semantic Media Ontology

The Semantic Media ontology, shown in Figure 1, is an application ontology that allows for describing media-specific device capabilities and related media content. A mobile device may be described as follows:

```
MobileDevice rdf:type SmartObject
MobileDevice acceptsMediaType Audio
MobileDevice  transmitsMediaType Audio
MobileDevice  hasMedia "file://media/groove.mp3"^^xsd:anyURI
MobileDevice rendersMediaAs Audio
```

The system configures itself through ontological reasoning based on these media type descriptions (as described in Section 6). A media player event of type `PlayEvent`, that would be generated when the mobile device starts playing music, is described as follows:

```
event1234-ABCD rdf:type PlayEvent
event1234-ABCD semint:inXSDDateTime "2001-10-26T21:32:52"^^xsd:dateTime
MobileDevice launchesEvent event1234-ABCD
```

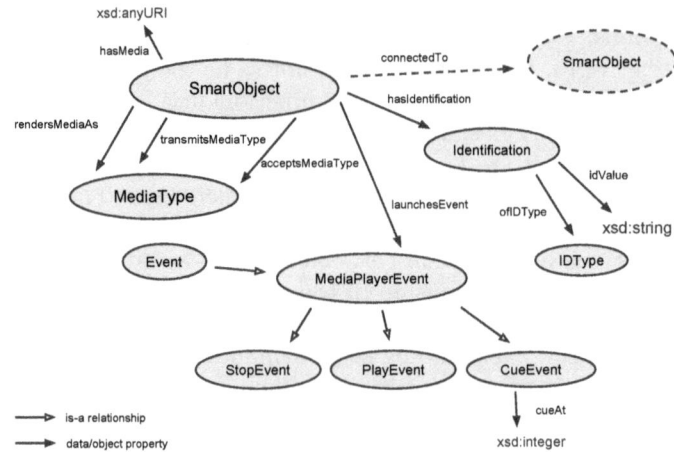

Fig. 1. Semantic Media Ontology

Smart objects may be connected to one another using the `connectedTo` relationship. When a device receives an event notification, it first verifies that it is currently connected to the device that generated the event, before responding to the event.

Smart objects may be connected to one another directly if there is a semantic match between transmitted and accepted media types. Otherwise a semantic transformer (introduced in the next section) will have to be be introduced to transform the shared content, while still preserving the actual meaning of the connection.

5   Semantic Transformers

The term *semantic transformers* is used in the context of the SOFIA project to refer to virtual devices that transform user actions into interaction events and perform matching and transformation of shared data and content. To this end, the work done for touch and pen-tablet interaction by the recently established W3C Web Events Working Group was taken as a starting point [1].

A semantic transformer is responsible for interpreting data coming from different smart objects and data sources into possible user goals, and maps them onto the plurality of available services. This facilitates a paradigm change from today's function-oriented interaction to a future of goal-oriented interaction.

User-action events are high-level input actions which capture and report the intention of the user's action directly, rather than just reporting the associated hardware input event that triggered the action. This high level of abstraction enables developers to write applications, which will work across different devices and services, without having to write specific code for each possible input device. The W3C Web Events Working Group defined four conceptual layers for interactions (for touch- and pen-tablet interaction) [1]:

physical. This is the lowest level, and deals with the physical actions that a user takes when interacting with a device, such as pressing a physical button.

gestural. This is a middle layer between the physical and representational layer, and describes specific mappings between the two; for example, a "pinch" gesture may represent the user placing two fingers on a screen and moving them together at the physical layer. This may map to a "zoom-in" event at the representational layer.

representational. This is the highest level of abstraction in the event model, and indicates the means by which the user is performing a task, such as zooming in, panning, navigating to the next page, activating a control, etc.

intentional. This layer indicates the intention of the task a user is trying to perform, such as viewing more or less detail (zooming in and out), viewing another part of the larger picture (panning), and so forth.

Table 1. Examples of representational events in a smart environment

Representational Event	Entity this event can be performed on
AdjustLevel	Volume, Lighting
switchOnOff	Lighting, any SmartObject
Navigate	Playlist, Menu, SequentialData
Undo/Redo	Any interaction event
Stop/Start	Application, Media
DragAndDrop	Media
Query	Media, other events

In Table 1 examples of possible representational events are defined. A representational event has more than one possible entity that it can be performed on, as well as more than one possible entity that triggers it, i.e., there exists some ambiguity. Only when no ambiguity exists as to which entity it is performed on, as well as the action which the user is trying to accomplish, we refer to it as an intentional event. Semantic transformations occur between physical actions (such as pressing a button or doing a gesture) and representational events, as well as between representational events and intentional events.

Building on the semantic transformers as they are applied to user actions, they can also be used to map and transform shared content between smart objects. The next section describes how this can be achieved.

6   Implementation

We illustrate our implementation of semantic transformers by means of a use case scenario, where the semantic transformers were introduced as part of a smart home pilot (as defined in the SOFIA project). In this use case scenario, media content is shared among several devices in a smart home setting. Music can be shared between a mobile device, a stereo speaker set (connected to the smart space through a Sound/Light KP) and a lighting device that can render the mood of the music with coloured lighting.

In the use case scenario, a Bonding Device [4] renders these light effects, but it accepts only RGB values, and cannot render music directly. The Bonding Device, created by Philips Research Eindhoven, provides a means to connect friends and siblings living apart, allowing them to share experiences, and stay in touch in a new way. The Bonding Device consists of two identical devices that enable indirect communication between relatives or friends at remote locations, by means of detecting human presence and activity at one side, and rendering this information at the other side, to establish a feeling of social connectedness. It responds to both implicit and explicit behavior of the user, e.g. when a Bonding Device detects the presence of a person and his/her proximity to the device, this information is rendered with particular light patterns at the remote side. Additionally it can render lighting effects to communicate the mood of music played by the friend or sibling at one side of the Bonding Device, and have the lighting effects mirrored on the remote Bonding Device.

The Bonding Device is described using the Semantic Media ontology as:

```
BondingDevice rdf:type SmartObject
BondingDevice acceptsMediaType RGBValues
BondingDevice rendersMediaAs Lighting
```

For the implementation of semantic transformers we consider the following scenario: "Mark and Dries start listening to music on a mobile device. They wish to render the music on a lighting device for some visual effects. They establish a semantic connection between the mobile device and the Bonding Device and the light effects are rendered on the Bonding Device."

The Bonding Device accepts dynamic lighting information in the form of a stream of RGB values. What makes this scenario interesting is that the mobile device itself is not capable of transmitting these RGB values, but the Sound/Light KP (a virtual device in the smart space) is. The Sound/Light KP acts as a semantic transformer, converting the music stream generated by the mobile device into the RGB values required by the Bonding Device. From the user's point of view, the only *required* connection is that between the mobile device and the Bonding Device, while the smart space takes care of the rest.

The Sound/Light KP is described as follows:

```
SoundLightKP rdf:type SmartObject
SoundLightKP acceptsMediaType Audio
SoundLightKP transmitsMediaType RGBValues
SoundLightKP  hasIdentification id4321
id4321 ofIDType IPAddress
id4321 idValue "192.168.1.4:1234"
```

The stream of RGB values is sent via a separate TCP/IP connection, so the Bonding Device needs to know whether the source device is capable of communicating via TCP/IP. Since smart objects in the smart space can be identified using their IP address and port number, we can use the identification information to infer a `communicatesByTCPIP` data property that can be read by the Bonding Device. To relate the `SmartObject` directly to the `IDType`, we use a property chain:

$$\text{hasIdentification} \circ \text{ofIDType} \sqsubseteq \text{hasIDType}^5$$

We then infer the `communicatesByTCPIP` data property by specifying a `TCPIPObject` subclass:

```
Class: TCPIPObject
    EquivalentTo:
        hasIDType value IPAddress,
        communicatesbyTCPIP value true
    SubClassOf:
        SmartObject
```

In order to determine the media source for the bonding device, we first need to perform semantic matching of the media types. We first define `isAccepted-MediaTypeOf` as the inverse property of `acceptsMediaType`, and then define the following property chain:

$$\text{transmitsMediaType} \circ \text{isAcceptedMediaTypeOf} \sqsubseteq \text{convertsMediaType}$$

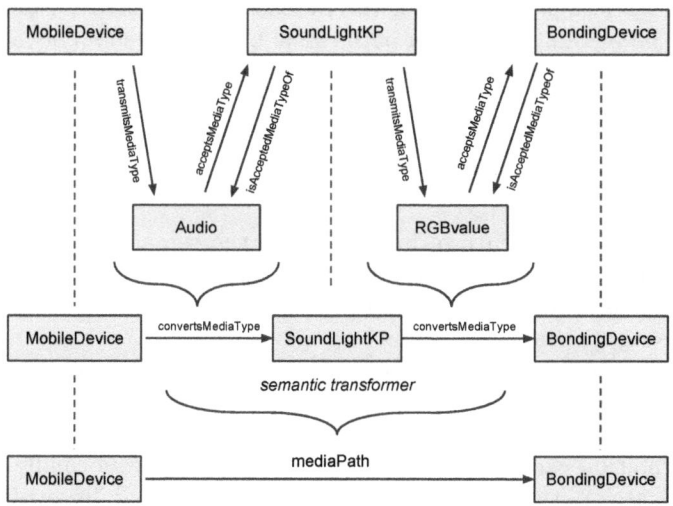

Fig. 2. Inferring the media path

---

⁵ The concatenation of two relations R and S is expressible by $R \circ S$, while $R \sqsubseteq S$ indicates that R is a subset of S.

This allows us to match media types between smart objects. We can then infer a *media path* between the mobile device and the Bonding Device with the Sound/Light KP acting as a semantic transformer using another property chain:

$$\text{convertsMediaType} \circ \text{convertsMediaType} \sqsubseteq \text{mediaPath}$$

To then determine the media source itself we have to use SWRL (Semantic Web Rule Language)[6], as the expressivity of OWL does not allow for inferring the media source if there are more than one `convertsMediaType` relationship linked to the Bonding Device:

`convertsMediaType(?x1,?x2)` $\wedge$ `convertsMediaType(?x2,?x3)` $\Rightarrow$ `mediaSourceSO(?x3, ?x2)`

We can also infer whether a device is a Semantic Transformer or not using:

```
Class: SemanticTransformer
    EquivalentTo:
        (canAcceptMediaTypeFrom some SmartObject) and
        (convertsMediaType some SmartObject)
    SubClassOf:
        SmartObject
```

The end result is that the Bonding Device responds to the mobile device's media events (based on the Semantic Connections `connectedTo` relationship), but uses the Sound/Light KP as a media source for generating dynamic lighting. The `connectedTo` relationship between the mobile device and the Bonding Device should only be possible if a media path exists between the two devices. Figure 2 illustrates the entire process of inferring the media path from the original media type definitions.

7   Conclusion

Judging from the experience of implementing the semantic transformers, such an approach to solving interoperability problems appears promising. In simple use cases, we found that the mechanisms developed and presented in this paper show promising results.

Using the the *Semantic Media Ontology*, we were able to define a smart object in terms of the media types it accepts and transmits. Based on these descriptions, semantic transformers can be used to transform media types in order to enable information exchange between devices that would normally not be able to communicate. With only a minimal set of device capabilities described, the system is able to perform self-configuration using ontological reasoning.

Acknowledgment. SOFIA is funded by the European Artemis programme under the subprogramme SP3 Smart environments and scalable digital service.

---

[6] http://www.w3.org/Submission/SWRL/

References

1. W3C Web Events Working Group Charter,
   http://www.w3.org/2010/webevents/charter/
2. OWL web ontology language use cases and requirements (2004),
   http://www.w3.org/TR/webont-req
3. Chen, H., Perich, F., Finin, T., Joshi, A.: SOUPA: standard ontology for ubiquitous and pervasive applications. In: Mobile and Ubiquitous Systems: Networking and Services, MOBIQUITOUS 2004, pp. 258–267 (2004)
4. Dadlani, P., Markopoulos, P., Kaptein, M., Aarts, E.: Exploring connectedness and social translucence in awareness systems. In: CHI 2010 Workshop on Designing and Evaluating Affective Aspects of Sociable Media to Support Social Connectedness, Atlanta, GA, USA, April 10-15 (2010)
5. Feijs, L., Hu, J.: Component-wise mapping of media-needs to a distributed presentation environment. In: The 28th Annual International Computer Software and Applications Conference (COMPSAC 2004), pp. 250–257. IEEE Computer Society, Hong Kong (2004)
6. Hu, J., Feijs, L.M.G.: IPML: Extending Smil for Distributed Multimedia Presentations. In: Zha, H., Pan, Z., Thwaites, H., Addison, A.C., Forte, M. (eds.) VSMM 2006. LNCS, vol. 4270, pp. 60–70. Springer, Heidelberg (2006)
7. Hu, J., Feijs, L.: Ipml: Structuring distributed multimedia presentations in ambient intelligent environments. International Journal of Cognitive Informatics & Natural Intelligence (IJCiNi) 3(2), 37–60 (2009)
8. Ngo, H.Q., Shehzad, A., Liaquat, S., Riaz, M., Lee, S.-Y.: Developing Context-Aware Ubiquitous Computing Systems with a Unified Middleware Framework. In: Yang, L.T., Guo, M., Gao, G.R., Jha, N.K. (eds.) EUC 2004. LNCS, vol. 3207, pp. 672–681. Springer, Heidelberg (2004)
9. Niezen, G., van der Vlist, B., Hu, J., Feijs, L.: From events to goals: Supporting semantic interaction in smart environments. In: IEEE Symposium on Computers and Communications, ISCC 2010, June 22-25, pp. 1029–1034 (2010)
10. Villalonga, C., Strohbach, M., Snoeck, N., Sutterer, M., Belaunde, M., Kovacs, E., Zhdanova, A.V., Goix, L.W., Droegehorn, O.: Mobile Ontology: Towards a Standardized Semantic Model for the Mobile Domain. In: Di Nitto, E., Ripeanu, M. (eds.) ICSOC 2007. LNCS, vol. 4907, pp. 248–257. Springer, Heidelberg (2009)
11. van der Vlist, B., Niezen, G., Hu, J., Feijs, L.: Design semantics of connections in a smart home environment. In: Chen, L.-L., Djajadiningrat, T., Feijs, L.M.G., Kyffin, S., Steffen, D., Young, B. (eds.) Proceedings of Design and Semantics of Form and Movement (DeSForM 2010), Koninklijke Philips Electronics N.V., Lucerne, Switzerland, pp. 48–56 (2010)
12. van der Vlist, B., Niezen, G., Hu, J., Feijs, L.: Semantic connections: Exploring and manipulating connections in smart spaces. In: 2010 IEEE Symposium on Computers and Communications (ISCC), June 22-25, pp. 1–4 (2010)
13. Weiser, M.: The computer for the 21st century. Scientific American (September 1991)

TV-kiosk: An Open and Extensible Platform for the Wellbeing of an Ageing Population

Maarten Steenhuyse, Jeroen Hoebeke, Ann Ackaert,
Ingrid Moerman, and Piet Demeester

Ghent University – IBBT, Department of Information Technology (INTEC),
Gaston Crommenlaan 8 Bus 201, 9050 Ghent, Belgium
`firstname.lastname@intec.ugent.be`

Abstract. The ageing population is becoming a growing challenge to society. User-centered ICT solutions adapted to elderly can play a prime role in dealing with these challenges. This paper presents TV-kiosk, an open and extensible TV-based platform that aims to stimulate social interaction, avoid isolation and deliver information. One of its distinguishing features is the underlying decentralized network communication approach based on advanced technology to securely and automatically interconnect devices and the TV-based user interface specifically designed for elderly. The openness and extensibility of the platform make it possible to easily integrate all kinds of new and existing e-services. Currently, a field trial is ongoing in a care center where TV-kiosk is being used by elderly, their family and caregivers.

Keywords: Elderly people, e-services, well-being, TV, platform, network virtualization, decentralized.

1 Introduction

ICT is continuously evolving at a very fast pace and plays an ever increasing role in our daily life. Technologies such as the Internet, mobile phones, social networks, interactive digital TV, etc. have become an indispensable part of our life, but not of everybody's life. Despite their popularity, these ICT technologies have not yet strongly penetrated into the daily life of many elderly. The majority of them is not computer literate, which make them digital outsiders for the current web applications and digital devices that are frequently used by their relatives.

This observation conflicts with the fact that innovation can enhance their quality of life, can help to cut the high costs that come with the ageing population and can create new business opportunities. Although there is a clear need, large opportunities and important role for ICT technologies to support the life of these people and to improve society, the reality is still different. However, the last few years, a lot of initiatives are trying to bridge this gap by designing ICT solutions specifically tailored to elderly and applying multi-disciplinary design methodologies in order to increase the accessibility and acceptance by the target group.

In this paper, we present such an initiative, TV-kiosk, which is the result of several years of cross-disciplinary research and which aims to stimulate social interaction,

M. Rautiainen et al. (Eds.): GPC 2011 Workshops, LNCS 7096, pp. 54–63, 2012.

avoid isolation and deliver information in a way adapted to elderly. The paper is structured as follows. In section 2, we describe in more detail the challenges we want to address and the requirements and assumptions we have put forward for the design of our platform. Section 3 describes the advanced networking technology behind the platform, whereas section 4 gives an overview of the services that have been designed and deployed. In section 5, we briefly describe the ongoing field trial of TV-kiosk in a care center, where the platform is being used by our target group, their family and caregivers. An analysis of the platform and comparison with related work in this field is subject of sections 6 and 7. Finally, section 8 concludes this paper.

2   Problem Statement and Approach

The ageing population is becoming a growing challenge to society in the industrialized world. By 2020, a quarter of Europe's population will be aged over 65 years. By 2050, people aged between 65 and 79 will make up almost a third. At the same time, the pool of potential caregivers is shrinking. New ICT technologies can help to meet the challenges of an ageing population in several areas. They can help them to carry out daily activities, to stimulate their social participation, to monitor their health, to facilitate social inclusion, to avoid isolation and loneliness or to enhance independent living.

In practice, the majority of elderly people does not yet enjoy the benefits of digitalization for several reasons. There is the age-related decline in cognitive functions, which has a profound effect on the capabilities of elderly in using new technologies [1]. The current interface design does not match these cognitive capabilities, and is sometimes even difficult for technology-prone people [2]. Last but not least, there is the overall acceptance of technologies based on issues such as control, trust, privacy, dignity or usability [3]. As such, designing new technologies is a problem with many facets, requiring multi-disciplinary efforts crossing the entire development spectrum and involving all stakeholders [4].

In this paper, we will focus on two important areas where ICT can make an important contribution: social inclusion and information access. Elderly are vulnerable to social isolation and have less access to information. Family and friends often have a busy life or live at distant locations, not having time for regular visits. However, social interaction with family and friends is important for their wellbeing and health. Within a care setting, caregivers spent a lot of time on administrative tasks, already reducing the time they can spend on their core task, providing care to people. With the decrease of workforce in the healthcare sector, this problem will become even more prevalent. However, access to information about the world and the environment they live (e.g. care center) in is important, offering a window to the world and helping to feel connected with society.

For these areas we wanted to realize a user centered ICT platform, usable by elderly people not acquainted with ICT technologies at all. At the same time, it had to address the above issues related to the acceptance and accessibility of new ICT technologies by following a multi-disciplinary design methodology. Next to this, we outlined a number of other requirements and assumptions that have driven the design of the platform. If we look at a Flemish study on the use of digital media by elderly, we can observe that TV is most popular [5]. This suggests that TV is an attractive medium to provide ICT solutions usable by the target group with little training. As such, the TV set was chosen as a primary interaction screen for the elderly, a PC or laptop for the other involved actors. To interconnect all actors securely over the Internet and to share and discover services, a secure, flexible and self-organizing solution was needed, hiding all underlying technological complexity. For the platform, we had several services in mind within our two target areas, but we wanted the platform to be extensible and open as well. Extensible, in order to be able to include other services - addressing other areas relevant to an ageing population - that could be deployed according to evolving needs of the users or in order to be able to integrate existing Internet-based services within the simplified user interface. Open, in order to allow other parties to design new services for the platform, which could lead to new and innovative services and accelerate the uptake of the solution.

Based on the above requirements and assumptions, the TV-kiosk platform was built, which will be further presented in the following sections.

3   The Technology

As stated, we require a secure, flexible and self-organizing solution in order to interconnect all actors (e.g. elderly, family, caregivers) over the Internet. In order to have an open and extensible service platform, we have chosen not to adopt a centralized solution controlled by a single service provider as is mostly being done. Instead, we have used our Virtual Private Ad-Hoc Network (VPAN) platform which combines ad hoc networking, peer-to-peer techniques and ubiquitous computing aspects to realize communication between trusted groups of devices [6].

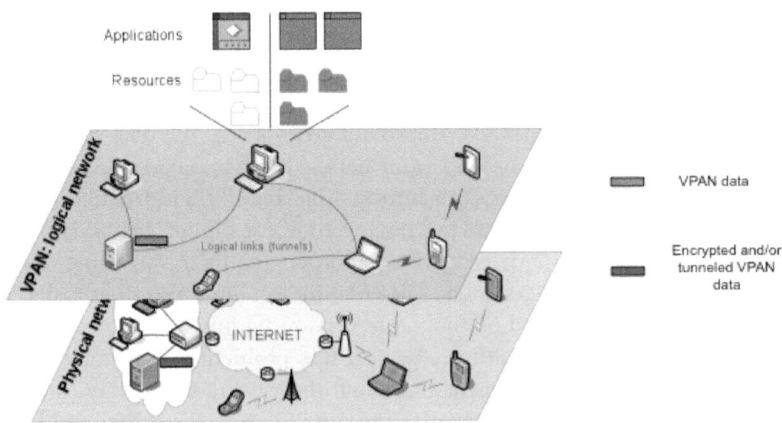

Fig. 1. Virtual Private Ad-Hoc Network concept

Through this VPAN technology, multiple devices at distant locations that need secure and easy access to each other's data and services are fully automatically and securely grouped in a logical, virtual network, regardless of the heterogeneity of underlying networks. Based on security information, devices can verify if they are member of the same group, after which they can setup secure connections to exchange information. The virtual network will organize and maintain itself, regardless of the devices' location, temporary interruptions in connectivity or upon mobility. No user interaction is required. The technology also contains a service framework that automatically announces the availability of shared services to other members of the same group and allows user-friendly access and management. Any service can be deployed on top of the logical network. For more details on the VPAN platform we refer to [7].

As such, the VPAN technology effectively hides the technological complexity of the interconnection between devices and is able to create permanent and closed groups. Furthermore, the technology meets the flexibility requirements, not only in terms of devices and services, but a device can also be member of multiple groups, which are all nicely shielded from each other.

Figure 2 illustrates how the VPAN technology is now being used in the TV-Kiosk platform. Secure and separated VPANs allow users to easily interact with each other. The "Home for the Elderly" VPAN offers services related to the care center. All residents are member of this group. On the other hand, every resident can be member of a private (for his family) "Family" VPAN, which allows family members to offer services such as photo sharing from their home.

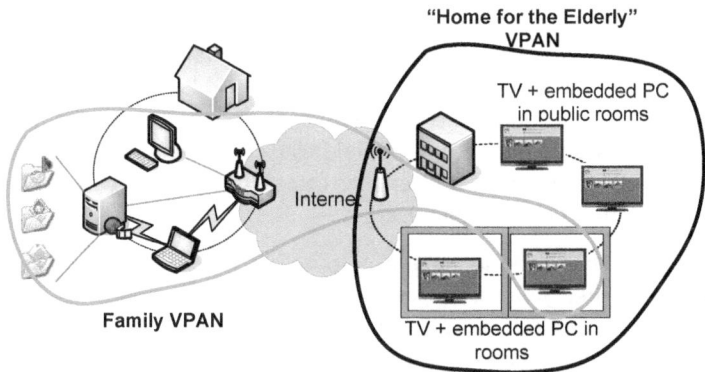

Fig. 2. Family and elderly home VPANs

4   The Services

On top of the networking and service discovery functionality offered by VPAN, we developed an accessible user interface for elderly on their TV. With a simple remote control users can access the service of choice in a few steps. To keep navigation simple, the remote has as few buttons as possible; a home button enables them to return to the start screen at any time. The start screen corresponds with the groups (i.e. VPANs) the user is member of.

Figure 3 depicts schematically where the content can originate from in our prototype setup. Next to content delivered using VPAN networks it is also possible to access Internet services on condition these are simple, preferably tailored with the target group in mind, and being integrated in the user interface. To enable extensibility, a plugin system has been used to implement the services and easily allow the creation of new services. In the following paragraphs we elaborate further on the design requirements we considered and the developed services.

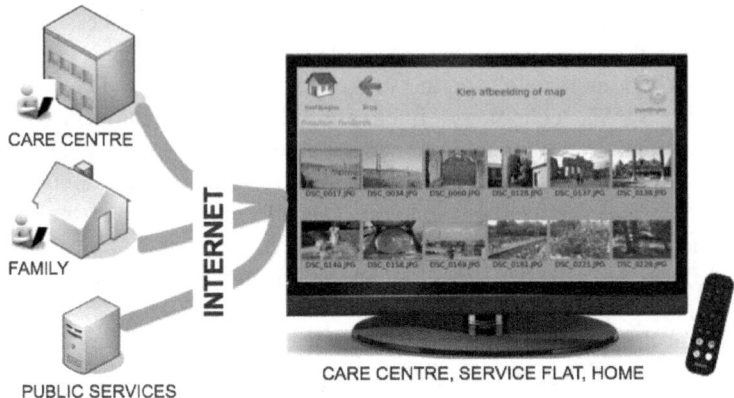

Fig. 3. The TV-Kiosk prototype

As mentioned before, in order to reach the target group, technological complexity must be hidden as much as possible. To this end, we collaborated closely with usability experts, people in the field such as care providers and last but not least the targeted end users. Development took place in different phases, collecting feedback obtained through usability research and setting up field trials to improve the product and obtain a satisfactory final result. For the user interfaces, the following usability guidelines have been taken into account during design:

- User Interfaces should be as simple as possible. The more information a screen holds, the more likely the user gets confused. A better approach is to use more screens than to try to fit everything on one screen.
- User interaction should be as simple as possible. Interaction choices should be kept at a minimum. Regular keyboards and mouse are usually inappropriate for the targeted users.
- The user should be guided as much as possible. A tutorial like interface is needed where every possible step is clearly explained.

Figure 4 shows the TV-Kiosk platform and some services in action. The top left picture shows the TV setup with the photo viewer service and the top right shows the music player. The screenshots at the bottom show how information can be displayed to the user, both for a VPAN service (activities in the care center) and a public Internet service (weather forecast).

For the service providers, such as staff in the care center and family members, a PC version of the software is available with plugins to share and/or create content. Next to this, we also built a web application that enables elderly to access messages and pictures posted by a relative using a Facebook plugin. This nicely illustrates how widely used web services can be easily integrated into our platform and complement our services running on top of the decentralized VPAN platform.

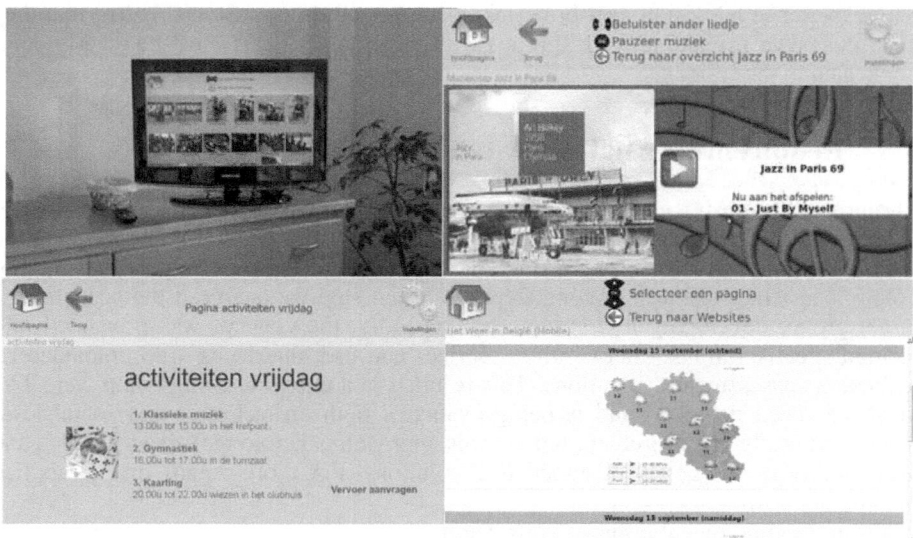

Fig. 4. Screenshots services

5   The Field Trial

We deployed the TV-Kiosk platform in a retirement home where three residents and family members were selected based on the mental fitness of the residents and the willingness to cooperate. We installed our system in the room of the residents and in a public room. We equipped a PC used by the staff with the PC version of our software. This PC acts as content provider for the services in the "Home for the Elderly" group, which maps to a VPAN on the networking level. Typical services involve information about the retirement home: planned activities, menu of the week, pictures of past activities, etc. The family members also installed the PC version of the software on their computer at home. This allowed them to create a "Family" group, enabling them to share pictures, music, messages and other content. Finally, a third group "External" is available which can be used for third-party providers that have an agreement with the retirement home to provide content. For example, a museum can provide pictures of the latest exhibitions.

During an initial field trial, TV-kiosk was tested, feedback collected and improvements were made. Currently a second field trial is ongoing using the enhanced version of our platform [8]. From this first field trial we have learned that a major motivation to participate was that the platform enables the residents and their relatives to have regular contact without the need to move to the retirement home. Despite the user-friendly television interface, some residents still have some difficulty using it and need assistance from staff or family. Furthermore, even family members sometimes lack the basic computer knowledge to manage the sharing of pictures and other content despite the user-friendly interface. Therefore, it is important to provide clear manuals and support. Also, the residents typically see a television as a passive medium. They have to get used to the active input required to access the information they want. Furthermore, they experience television as a broadcast medium and do not always realize that they have their own private network (group) with their family. This must be clearly communicated to the residents.

6   Requirement Analysis

Throughout the design and implementation of the TV-kiosk platform we have ensured to meet all the requirements we have put forward in the beginning. In cooperation with usability experts, we applied a user-centered multi-disciplinary design methodology consisting of the following steps. In a first step we analyzed the needs of the target group, developing a first concept. Secondly, the concept was translated into technological solutions – networking, services and user interfaces -, accompanied by technology assessment evaluations. This resulted in a third - ongoing - step were TV-kiosk has been deployed and is being evaluated both on technical and social level during two trials in a retirement home. This approach is key to realize acceptance and accessibility of the newly designed ICT solutions. For more details on the applied methodology, we refer to [9].

From a technological point of view, we have chosen to use the VPAN platform, allowing the creation of multiple secure and self-organizing virtual IP networks according to the users needs and on top of which any service can be deployed and run. Apart from a one-time configuration step, this technology succeeds in hiding all underlying complexity in securely interconnecting the devices used by the different actors and automatically discovering shared services.

By taking a decentralized communication approach, opposed to centralized solutions, we avoid central control over the services that can be deployed and over the data exchanged or stored. In combination with an API to make use of the service discovery framework and to integrate services in the user interface as new plugins, any developer is able to create its own applications that can run within the logical VPAN networks, forming the basis of an open and easily extendable platform. Finally, next to the deployment of services within these virtual networks, we have also demonstrated the integration of existing Internet-based services within our simplified user interface. As such, our platform is capable of supporting both services running within the shielded logical networks as well as existing web-based services, combining the best of both worlds.

The above discussion reveals how TV-kiosk is capable of meeting the requirements and has taken precautions to ensure the accessibility of the technology. From the ongoing field trial, we are continuously collecting feedback that helps us to further improve the platform.

7   Related Work

There are some other efforts also targeted to elderly and aiming to avoid social isolation, to stimulate social interaction or to deliver information. In this section we will provide an overview of the most relevant work in these fields within Europe and will compare it with the approach taken by TV-kiosk. We will restrict ourselves to those initiatives that also make use of Internet for communication and of TV as the primary interaction screen, which is best suited for people not acquainted with ICT.

Within Europe there are several, both finished as well as ongoing, projects related to TV-kiosk, especially within the AAL Joint Programme. Table 1 gives an overview of the most important European initiatives.

Table 1. Related EU initiatives

Name	Short description and main characteristics
T-Seniority [10]	The T-seniority project (Expanding the Benefits of Information Society to Older People through Digital TV Channels) aims to build an online service platform that offers e-Care Services primarily via digital and digital interactive TV. A citizen or patient sitting in front of TV screen, with a remote control on hand, will be able to choose among many different options of public or personalized services. The services are deployed on the Internet using a Software as a Service model and is aimed to integrate many different services.
ALICE [11]	The ongoing ALICE project (Advanced Lifestyle Improvement system & new Communication Experience) recognizes social engagement with relatives and friends as an important determinant of quality of life. The overall objective is to research, develop and integrate a set of ICT-based services into the existing TV set allowing elderly people to enjoy experiences of communication and social interaction based on ICT and simplified access to Web resources. The system will consist of a set-top box connected to the TV and a remote control tailored to elderly. Also, an intuitive user interface will be developed allowing simple navigation and control. The final system should also offer services like personal alarming systems or health monitoring devices. A pilot installation is foreseen.
FoSIBLE [12]	The ongoing FoSIBLE project (Fostering Social Interactions for a Better Life of the Elderly) considers social interactions beyond the near environment with remotely living family members and friends to be equally important as social interaction within the neighborhood. Different applications will be developed and integrated in a TV-based Social Media Center. Also, issues related to usability, user acceptance and accessibility will be specifically addressed.
HOMEdot OLD [13]	The ongoing HOMEdotOLD project aims to provide a highly personalized, intuitive and open TV-based platform to advance the social interaction of elderly people, aiming to prevent isolation and loneliness. The architecture is centralized consisting of a set-top box and an external application server where the services reside.
Join-in [14]	The recently started Join-In project (Senior Citizens Overcoming Barriers by Joining Fun Activities) aims at providing technologies for elderly persons to participate in social activities such as games and exer-games and have fun via digital media. The Internet can also be accessed via TV, an interface the entire target group is well acquainted with, by offering set-top boxes. Design-based research will be used.

From Table 1 it is clear that similar initiatives exists that aim to design TV-based solutions for elderly in order to stimulate social interaction and avoid isolation. In many cases, the research methodology also explicitly focuses on usability and accessibility and field trials or pilots are seen as a crucial part of this process. It should be noted that, apart from T-Seniority, all projects have only recently started, not having published concrete results or mentioning to have reached a field trial phase. In that respect, TV-kiosk can be seen as one of the first initiatives that has succeeded in building a TV-based platform and evaluating it in a field trial. Therefore, these other initiatives strengthen our belief that a TV-based platform is a good approach to bring ICT technologies to elderly in view of user acceptance and accessibility.

When considering the services that are being offered or targeted, it should be noticed that some of the projects foresee a plethora of services, going beyond services currently offered by TV-kiosk, which primarily focus on social inclusion or dissemination of information. However, through our open and extensible design, we are confident to include more health-care related services in the future.

When looking at the technology behind the solutions, it can be said that, based on the publicly available information on the mentioned projects, the TV-kiosk approach is unique by taking a decentralized communication approach based on an advanced networking technology to securely and automatically interconnect devices both locally and over the Internet. The other solutions are centralized, where the offered services reside on a server. It is our belief that our decentralized approach has some interesting advantages, especially in view of the creation of an open and extensible platform for which anyone should be able to design novel services. However, we also have the possibility to integrate existing Internet services or centralized services, combining the best of both worlds, depending on the type of service being considered.

8   Conclusions and Future Work

It is clear that there is a strong need for ICT technologies tailored to elderly and designed in a cross-disciplinary way, starting from design up to field trial evaluation, in order to increase acceptance and accessibility. Hereby the fact that the majority of elderly is not computer literate and that there is an age-related decline in cognitive functions, impacting the capabilities in using new technologies, should be taken into account. Currently, several initiatives have emerged in Europe that recognize these issues and that start building solutions using TV as the prime interaction screen, since this is the medium elderly are most familiar with and are able to use with little training.

The TV-kiosk platform presented in this paper is one such an initiative for an ageing population that aims to stimulate social interaction, avoid isolation and deliver information. One of its distinguishing features is the underlying decentralized network communication approach based on advanced technology to securely and automatically interconnect devices and the user interface specifically adapted to elderly. The openness and extensibility of the platform make it possible to easily integrate all kinds of new and existing e-services. Next to this, a second field trial is already taking place, whereas most other initiatives have only recently started in designing and building TV-based solutions targeted to elderly.

Although a lot of research has been carried out already in order to create the platform, there is still a lot of room for additional research and extensions. For example, since government is stimulating the independent living of elderly, it is interesting to broaden our scope and extend our field trial in order to target also elderly living independently. New and more interactive e-services will be developed for this case such as the ordering of meals or the arrangement of transport. Also the extension with more health-related services such as monitoring needs to be considered. Such a wide variety of services on top of an open and extensible platform should result in a customizable system that can be easily deployed and extended according to the evolving needs of elderly. The advent of small and low-power sensors makes it interesting to extend our networking technology and platform in order to be able to incorporate sensors as well. Finally, as part of the cross-disciplinary approach, also the business aspect should be investigated, looking at all involved stakeholders and organizations in control of healthcare financing. This, in combination with the technology presented here is required to make such a platform a reality and contribute to a better and smarter society for an ageing population.

References

1. Slegers, K., van Boxtel, M.P.J., Jolles, J.: The Efficiency of Using Everyday Technological Devices by Older Adults: The Role of Cognitive Functions. Aeging and Society 29(2), 309–325 (2009)
2. Wilkowska, W., Ziefle, M., Arning, K.: Older Adults' Navigation Performance when Using Small-screen Devices: Does a Tutor Help? In: 9th International Conference on Work With Computer Systems, Beijing, China (2009)
3. Pew, R., Van Hemel, S.: Technology for Adaptive Aging. National Academies Press, Atlanta (2004)
4. Slegers, K.: Research Approaches into Communication Technologies for Older Users. In: CHI - Workshop Age Matters: Bridging the Generation Gap through Technology-mediated Interaction, Boston (2009)
5. Verté, D., De Donder, L.: Schaakmat of aan Zet? Monitor voor Lokaal Ouderenbeleid in Vlaanderen, Vandenbroele (2007)
6. Hoebeke, J., Holderbeke, G., Moerman, I., Dhoedt, B., Demeester, P.: Virtual Private Ad Hoc Networking. Wireless Personal Communications 38(1), 125–141 (2006)
7. Hoebeke, J.: Adaptive Ad Hoc Routing and its Application to Virtual Private Ad Hoc Networks. Ph.D. thesis, Ghent University (2007)
8. TV-kiosk Press Conference, http://www.smartcareplatform.eu/content/tv-kiosk-press-conference
9. Ackaert, A., Jacobs, A., Veys, A., Derboven, J., Van Gils, M., Buysse, H., Agten, S., Verhoeve, P.: A Multi-disciplinary Approach towards the Design and Development of Value+ eHomeCare Services. In: Yogesan, K., Bos, L., Brett, P., Gibbons, M.C. (eds.) Handbook of Digital Homecare. Series in Biomedical Engineering, vol. 2, pp. 243–267. Springer, Heidelberg (2009)
10. Moumtzi, V., Farinos, J., Wills, C.: T-Seniority: an online service platform to assist independent living of elderly population. In: 2nd International Conference on Pervasive Technologies Related to Assistive Environments, Corfu, Greece (2009)
11. Advanced Lifestyle Improvement System and New Communication Experience, http://www.aal-alice.eu
12. Fostering Social Interactions for a Better Life of the Elderly, http://fosible.eu
13. Home Services Advancing the Social Interaction of Elderly People, http://www.homedotold.eu
14. Senior Citizens Overcoming Barriers by Joining Fun Activities, http://www.itfunk.org/docs/prosjekter/AAL-Join-In.htm

Design of Easy Access Internet Browsing System for Elderly People Based on Android

Geng Li[1], Yuping Zhao[1], Bingli Jiao[1], and Timo Korhonen[2]

[1] Satellite & Wireless Communication Laboratory, Peking University,
Beijing, China
ligeng66@yahoo.com.cn, {yuping.zhao,jiaobl}@pku.edu.cn
[2] Department of Communications and Networking, Aalto University,
Espoo, Finland
timo.korhonen@tkk.fi

Abstract. In these years, the living quality of elderly is drawing more and more attention. In order to meet their needs for Internet we have designed tailored easy access Internet browser for tablet computers. The system integrates wireless network connection with the new Internet browser, and runs on Android OS which is currently widely used on tablet computers. Our pilot run with elderly verifies that the design indeed offers easier and convenient browsing experience.

Keywords: Elderly care, Internet browsing system, Android, tablet computers.

1 Introduction

Aging is one of the most important issues of 21st century. As a result, living quality of elderly draws also increasing attention. There is a large number of elderly who have a need to surf the Internet. As indicated by Czaja (1996), not much attention has focused on older Internet users until recently [1]. As the Internet develops and the number of websites increases, website designers have begun to focus on the needs of elderly. During the 18th International Conference of World Wide Web, an Internet expert said: "The elderly will become the fastest-growing class of network population."

Indeed, the network, full of all kinds of resources, will provides these people with enormous information, great convenience, abundant entertainments and close connections to their families. There is a study which demonstrates that aged adults who learn to use the Internet to search for information can experience a surge of activity in key decision-making and reasoning regions of the brain [2]. This is based on neuro-plasticity where other brain areas can take tasks of damaged areas. It was noted in another research that elderly who are more socially active and not as easily distressed, do not develop dementia as easily as the one who are distressed or socially Isolated [3]. Surfing the Internet provides the elderly with opportunities to develop their intellectual capacities, expand social network, and achieve a feeling of satisfaction, competency and self-esteem.

A traditional way to approach the Internet is by using personal computers. However, for elderly who are not familiar with computers, Internet becomes too exclusive.

M. Rautiainen et al. (Eds.): GPC 2011 Workshops, LNCS 7096, pp. 64–72, 2012.

For instance, a large number of elderly people can not handle the mouse easily. They have no idea about the scroll wheel and "double click". The pointer arrow on the screen can also be too small to find or track for elderly. And when interacting with websites, older users need to handle various computer interfaces not originally designed for them [4]. What's more, the immovability is also one of disadvantages of personal computers. Especially for the elderly, sitting in front of the computer for a longer time is definitely not an entertainment. Personal computers do not naturally fit well in ergonomic sense for a larger group of aged people.

Over the last decade, tablet computers have developed rapidly in software and hardware perspectives. Far and away, the best thing in tablet PCs is their mobility. They are lighter than laptops and support usually wireless connectivity which can enable WLAN, Bluetooth, and even 3G cellular networking. The user interface personalization, flat working surface and electronic input leverage simplify the controls of the tablet computers. Another advantage of tablet PCs over regular laptops is that the users don't lose any significant functionality when compared to tabletops. Although the average processing speed of tablet computers is generally slower for some big programs to run, they are fast enough to meet the need of most elderly.

In spite of the conveniences mentioned, there are still some other barriers in elderly Internet access. Setting up the access itself can be difficult. For instance, multiple menus can in effect hide the complex networking setups. Also, the existing Internet browsers can be too complex and often contain way too many function keys, most of which can be useless for them. In other words, the existing tablet computers and browsers can be much too difficult for elderly to conveniently surf the Internet.

Lack of experience and support makes it likely that elderly will have negative user experience. This can be a significant factor in computer anxiety [5]. Conversely, more encouraging user experience should foster a more positive attitude toward computers. Therefore, to overcome these barriers, our research aims to develop truly easy and fast Internet browsing system targeted especially to elderly.

2   Android Operating System

Android is a mobile operating system which is developed by Android Inc and now marketed by Google. As announced, Android is a truly open mobile platform. The Android platform is licensed under one of the most progressive open-source licenses available, giving operators and manufacturers unprecedented freedom to design, build and distribute own products [6]. A researcher predicted that Android will become in the very near future the most popular operating system framework for smart phones and tablet PCs.

Tablet computers with Android operating system are as such already quite easy to handle. There are three important keys in Android: Home, Back and Menu. When the Home key is pressed, user is returned to the desktop. When the Back key is pressed, return to the last activity or picture is made. When the Menu key is pressed, an optional menu will pop up. Except for these three keys, all the other controls can be accessed via a touch screen. There is a research indicating that touch screen and handwriting recognition are better than mouse and keyboard in browsing time, and touch screen is also found to be better in terms of performance time for keyword searches when compared to mouse or voice input. Also, it is more error free in keyword searcher [4]. These are the reasons why we have chosen Android to the development platform.

3   System Description

In order to provide the elderly a convenient Internet browsing experience, we integrate the WiFi settings and Internet browser. Our system is characterized by user interface simplicity, reduced number of menu keys, and clear and simple navigation paths. System applies a larger font size. However, the browser still contains all the basic functionalities of conventional browsers. Frequently visited websites can be memorized. The system is easy to learn and use.

"Activity" is a basic component of the Android systems, and the activities can be activated in sequence (Fig. 1.). Our system program consists of six activities. Generally, activities can run in parallel, still only one of them is displayed on the screen. However, in our system activation of some new activity will turn off the old one for easy management and power savings.

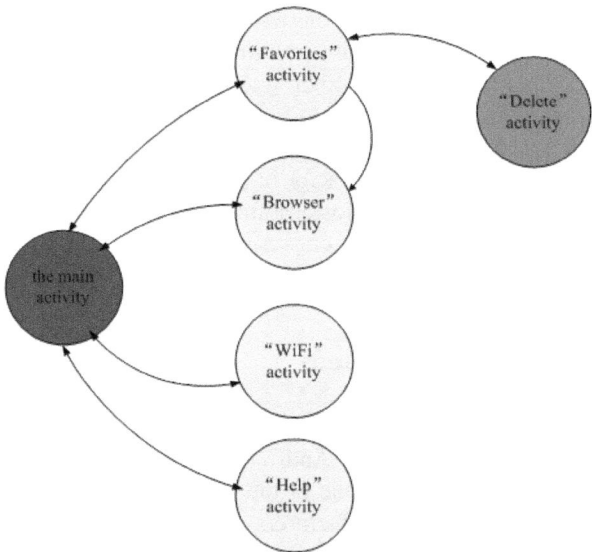

Fig. 1. System framework

The main activity is started when the system is initialized. The main interface contains four buttons, each of which represents a function. When the button is pressed, the corresponding activity is started. The main interface is shown in Fig. 2. When the Menu key is pressed, a menu containing two items will pop up, as shown in Fig. 3. The left item is "Settings", which guides the user to system setup, such as the language, input method, and so on. The right one is "Exit", which executes system exit.

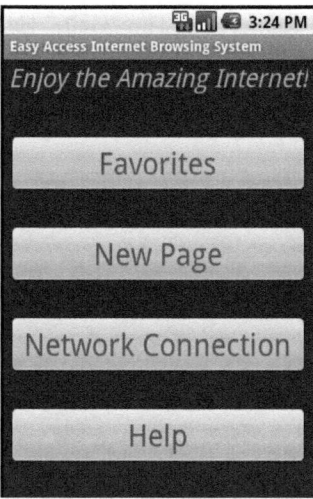

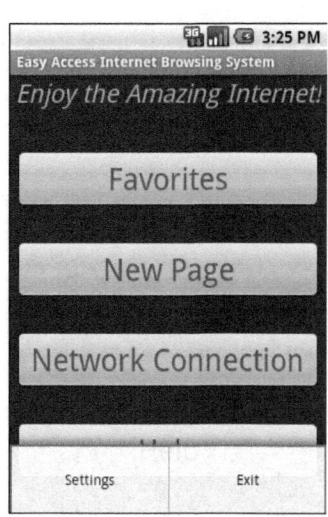

Fig. 2. The main interface   Fig. 3. Menu in the main interface

The "Favorites" activity is an item list and the label on each item is a name of website. When any item is pressed, the "Browser" activity is started. It will go to the corresponding website that the users selected earlier. The "Browser" activity can also be started by pressing the "New Page" button in the main interface.

The menu in the "Favorites" activity contains three items (Fig. 4). The "Home" item returns to the main interface and the "Exit" item shuts down the system. When the "Delete" item is pressed, the "Delete" activity will be started, as shown in Fig. 5. Users can delete any websites in the favorites. The list in this activity can be refreshed constantly.

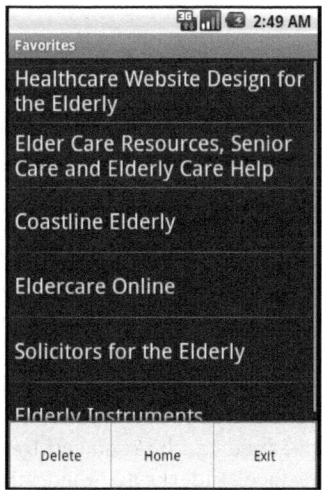

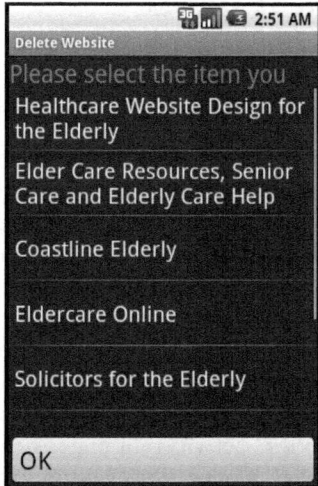

Fig. 4. Menu in Favorites   Fig. 5. Delete activity

The "WiFi" activity is used to setup the WiFi connection. The "Help" activity is a text window containing help items. The "WiFi" and "Help" activities as shown in Fig. 6 and Fig. 7 are started by pressing the "Network Connection" and "Help" buttons in the main interface, respectively.

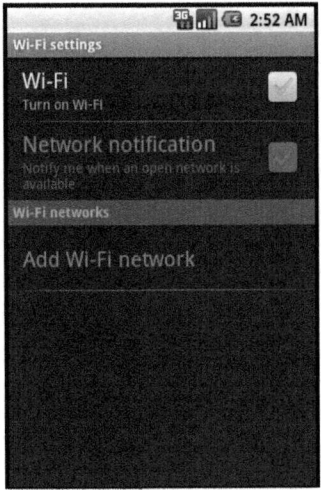

Fig. 6. WiFi activity

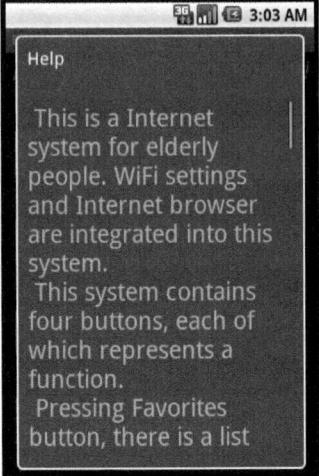

Fig. 7. Help activity

Our WiFi setup and the Internet browser deviate from the conventional Android approach that we inspect next.

4   Key Features

4.1   WiFi Settings

It is required to have network access to surf the Internet. For the wireless devices like tablet computers, WiFi is the most common way. To connect the wireless network, user needs to turn on the WiFi first, where after hot spots can be potentially joined. If the access is deciphered, a password is required. It is impossible to connect automatically for the first time. Users need to enter the WiFi Settings page and make a manual setup. In the conventional Android operating system, the WiFi setup requires going through the sequence: "Menu key→ Settings→ Wireless Settings→ WiFi Settings", which is obviously quite difficult to manage for elderly.

Activities correspond to a Java class. "WiFi Settings" is an inner class which is already defined in the system library. This needs to be called by the system (it is attached to the "WiFi" activity). In our system, actions described can be replaced by pressing the"Network Connection" button in the main interface. Elderly can therefore set the

WiFi very easily and rapidly. In case if some elderly has no understanding about WiFi or network in general, the connection can be configured at first, and as long as the WiFi environment doesn't change, the network will be connected automatically afterward.

4.2 Favorites

The items in "Favorites" are saved in a writeable database, so the users can define favorites by themselves. The data management of Android applies SQLite, which is an open source embedded database engine. For its advantages of small core, fast and high efficiency, stability, reliability, portability and so on, SQLite is arguably the most widely deployed SQL database engine in the world.

A SQLite database is just a file stored in the /data/data/packagename/databases directory in the Android system [7]. A database file can have any number of tables. A table consists of columns, each of which has a name and a data type. To define these tables and column names, the program has to run Data Definition Language (DDL) statements at first. In this system, we create a table with four columns and the statement is shown as follows.

```
create table mytable (
_id integer primary key autoincrement,
time integer,
name text,
address text );
```

The "_id" column is designated as the PRIMARY KEY, a number that uniquely identifies the row. AUTOINCREMENT means that the database will add 1 to the key for every record to make sure it's unique [7]. The "time" column is for saving the time information. The items in the list will display in the order of time. The "name" column is for saving the name of each websites which shows on the label of the corresponding item. The "address" column is for saving the address of each websites. The browser can go directly to the website with the saved address.

4.3 Browser

The conventional browsers contain a large number of features and plug-heavyweights. Elderly who prefer easy access, the attractive graphical interface as such is not the major preference. So, the conventional browsers are not most suitable for them [8]. Therefore, we designed a new Internet browser based on Webkit library. As an open-source browser engine with a higher speed, less memory and other notable features, Webkit is found in Google Chrome, the Apple iPhone, and the Safari desktop browser but with a twist. With Webkit library, the Android system lets developers use the browser as a component right inside the application [9].

The browser of our system contains address bar and three basic navigation keys. The interface is simple and clear. As shown in Fig. 8, when the user presses the address bar, a soft keyboard will pop up. After typing the url address, the soft keyboard will cancel and the website will display. Whether entering from the favorites or by typing address

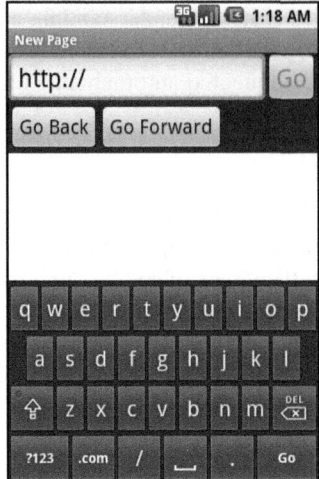
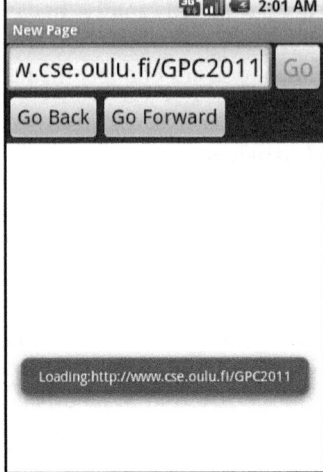

Fig. 8. Soft keyboard   **Fig. 9.** Prompt message

directly, a prompt message will be displayed prior entering the website, as shown in Fig. 9. Considering that a large number of people having presbyopia in older age, text on the buttons, address bar and also in the websites should show up in a much larger size than in conventional browsers that we have also implemented.

5   Evaluations and Results

WiFi access is available currently in some hot spots in China, such as community centers, district offices, public libraries, post offices, and voluntary agencies. We conducted a simple test with a small scale of participants. There were 16 users 50–70 engaged in the experiment.

All participants began by filling out a general-information questionnaire concerning their personal characteristics including age, education, and past computer and internet experience. Depending on their information, participants were assigned into one of two groups (conventional system and our system), which contained the similar characteristics of participants. A tablet computer with our Chinese language version system was used for the experiment. Each participant was given a paper of instructions, depending on the type of system the participant was assigned. A brief practice session was then conducted to help the participants understand the operation of the system and the tasks to be performed. Following the practice, each participant performed two consecutive trials with four tasks in each trial. The tasks (Table 1) are the same in the two trials, but participants could not read the instructions in second trail. The participants were instructed to perform the tasks as quickly as possible in 3 minutes. We recorded how many tasks each participant had finished in each trail.

Table 1. Testing tasks

Number	Task
1	Connect wireless network.
2	Open Google search website from the favorites (the website has already been added to favorites).
3	Open the homepage of Yahoo by typing the address in a new page.
4	Add Yahoo to favorites.

The results were shown in Table 2. The numbers in the sheet represent the average numbers of tasks that one participant had finished.

Table 2. Results of the simple test

	Conventional system	Our system
Trail1	1.75	2.625
Trail2	1	2.5

6　Conclusion and Further Work

These evaluations demonstrated that in our system access was significantly more convenient than in the conventional system. In the first trails, with the detailed instructions, each participant finished almost one more tasks in average with our system. They could access the Internet easily and fast. Comparing the D-values of the two trails, we can figure that without the instructions, participants could achieve almost the same performance as in Trial 1, which means that the usage of our system seems to be indeed easier to learn for elderly.

Based on these results, our system is generally useful for elderly. However, results need to be interpreted with caution given that the data were collected under controlled conditions. Furthermore, the system needs to be tested with a larger number of participants.

For the next stage, we will do more tests. Considering the WiFi environment is not widely covered in China, we plan to change the network connection strategy optionally to into 3G too. The testing facility can be moved to parks or nursing houses where there is a true need for developed ease of access Internet technology. During the tests, we will collect advices and feedback in order to analyze the elderly surfing practices more deeply and try to further recognize user requirements. In aiming to ease Internet access for elderly, we are going to develop more tools which can offer greater convenience, and help functionalities, thus providing the elderly more comfortability and functionality in the wide world of today's Internet.

Acknowledgments. This project is financially supported by National Science Foundation of China (NSFC) under the project "User-centric Design of Ubiquitous Welfare and Safety Services and Supporting Technologies for China and Finland".

References

1. Czaja, S.J.: Aging and the acquisition of computer skills. Aging and skilled performance: Advances in theory and applications, pp. 201–220 (1996)
2. Diabetes, U.: News update. Working with Older People 13, 5–10 (2009)
3. Gold, E.: Dementia and Neuroplasticity: What Might Help Today? Mental.help.net, http://www.mentalhelp.net/poc/view_doc.php?type=doc&id=29030&w=10&cn=231
4. Rau, P.L.P., Hsu, J.W.: Interaction devices and web design for novice older users. Educational Gerontology 31, 19–40 (2005)
5. Todman, J., Drysdale, E.: Effects of qualitative differences in initial and subsequent computer experience on computer anxiety. Computers in Human Behavior 20, 581–590 (2004)
6. Hall, S.P., Anderson, E.: Operating systems for mobile computing. Journal of Computing Sciences in Colleges 25, 64–71 (2009)
7. Burnette, E.: Hello, Android: introducing Google's mobile development platform: Pragmatic Bookshelf (2008)
8. Lam, J., Lee, M.: Bridging the Digital Divide-The Roles of Internet Self-Efficacy Towards Learning Computer and the Internet among Elderly in Hong Kong, China, p. 266b (2005)
9. Hongcan, Y., et al.: The design and realization of the Linux browser based on Webkit, pp. 188–191 (2010)

Exploring Pervasive Service Computing Opportunities for Pursuing Successful Ageing

Jiehan Zhou[1,2], Xiang Su[1], Mika Ylianttila[1], and Jukka Riekki[1]

[1] Computer Science and Engineering Laboratory and Infotech Oulu,
90014 University of Oulu, Finland
firstname.familyname@ee.oulu.fi
[2] Middleware Systems Research Group, Department of Electrical and Computer Engineering,
University of Toronto, Canada

Abstract. Pervasive Service Computing for Elderly applies service composition and pervasive computing into assisting elderly Activities of Daily Life. Taking advantages of context-awareness and service-oriented computing, Pervasive Service Computing expects to bring brilliant opportunities for pursuing global successful ageing. This paper proposes a Pervasive Service Computing for Elderly (PSC4E) framework for improving Quality of Life of elderly people, through providing being-, becoming-, and belonging-based services in context of population ageing trends, an elderly service provisioning model, and related studies.

Keywords: Pervasive computing, service computing, pervasive healthcare, elderly.

1 Introduction

Population ageing is a trend reflecting the increase in the number and proportion of elderly people in society. Population ageing implies a decline in the proportion of the population composed of children, and an increase in the proportion of elderly adults. Four major findings are given to population ageing in United National Human Development Report [8] as follows: 1) The world's number of elderly people is expected to exceed the number of children for the first time in 2045. 2) Population ageing results in universal reduction of productiveness. 3) Population ageing has major consequences and implications for all facets of human life. 4) Population ageing is enduring. The proportion of elderly has been rising steadily since 1950, passing from 8% in 1950 to 11% in 2009, and is expected to reach 22% in 2050. This paper cites age 65 as the entry point of becoming an elderly person. Ageing has a significant negative impact on society, including high caregiving costs, a growing burden to family caregivers [1], inadequate medical resources, and shortage of medical services in rural areas.

Successful ageing is regarded as an ultimate goal to address the ageing issue. Six dimensions of successful ageing are suggested in [2, 3] such as reduced physical disability over the age of 75, good self-ratings, greater length of normal life, etc.

M. Rautiainen et al. (Eds.): GPC 2011 Workshops, LNCS 7096, pp. 73–82, 2012.

Pursuing successful ageing has been targeted by adopting Information and Communication Technology (ICT) in the healthcare industry for years, in the name of pervasive healthcare computing [7], e-Inclusion [48], and Ambient Assisting Living (AAL) [49]. On-demand access to medical information anywhere and anytime has brought benefits to physicians and patients. More advanced applications like personal and assistive robotics can assist elderly persons and people with disabilities [4]. Efforts have also been made for facilitating elderly and disabled person's independence at home through smart environments [5][6]. Stanford [7] has pointed out that pervasive computing promises a significant improvement in quality of life for the elderly.

We consider successful ageing equal with independent ageing, that is, with the ability to complete basic daily activities without personal assistance. Pervasive Service Computing (PSC) aims to facilitate users' everyday activities by ubiquitously supporting them with network-accessed web services [13][19]. We believe that Pervasive Service Computing can improve independent ageing by delivering personal services that match each elderly person's particular needs. The main contribution of this paper is shaping this vision to the concept of Pervasive Service Computing for Elderly (PSC4E). We emphasize PSC4E as an emerging technology for achieving successful ageing.

The remainder of the paper is organized as follows: Section 2 presents National Center for Medical Rehabilitation Research (NCMRR) elderly impairment model for research on the navigation of independent ageing. Section 3 reviews Quality of Life domains and indicators of independent ageing. Section 4 studies the PSC4E service model. Section 5 presents the PSC4E framework. Section 6 presents a brief literature review. Conclusions and discussions are drawn in section 7.

2   NCMRR Elderly Disability Model

The elderly commonly have conditions that limit their daily activities. The National Center for Medical Rehabilitation Research (NCMRR) [45] defines five overlapping research domains relevant to studying disability.

Pathophysiology refers to the aberration from normal physiological and developmental processes. Research focuses on cellular, structural, or functional events subsequent to injury, disease, or genetic abnormality.

Impairment is a loss or abnormality at the organ level. Such organ impairment may cause difficulties with movement, hearing, vision, or cognition.

Functional limitation refers to lack of ability to perform an action within the range of an organ system. Function is the performance of an action for which a person or thing is especially fitted or normally used.

Disability is defined as a limitation in fulfilling tasks to expected levels. Research focuses on the successful adaptations made by individuals with disabilities.

Societal limitation refers to lack of ability to perform societal activities. Research examines the effectiveness of different rehabilitation interventions with the societal institutions.

3   Quality of Life Domains and Indicators

The concept of independent ageing is receiving growing attention around the world. Independent ageing links to the quality of life (QOL) of the elderly. The Centre for Health Promotion at University of Toronto defines QOL as the degree to which a person enjoys the important possibilities of his or her life [9]. The QOL domains and indicators, which apply to both younger and elderly people, are:

Being domain includes the basic aspects of "who one is," and has three indicators: Physical Being, Psychological Being, and Spiritual Being. **Becoming domain** refers to the purposeful activities carried out to achieve personal goals, hopes, and wishes. The three indictors in this area are Practical Becoming, Leisure Becoming, and Growth Becoming. **Belonging domain** includes a person's fit with his/her environment, and has three indicators: Physical Belonging, Social Belonging, and Community Belonging. Table 1 presents these three domains' indicators.

Table 1. Quality of life indicators

Indicator	Specification
physical being	physical health, personal hygiene, general physical appearance
psychological being	psychological health, self-esteem, self-concept and self-control
spiritual being	personal values, personal standards of conduct, spiritual beliefs
practical becoming	domestic activities, meeting health or social needs
leisure becoming	activities that promote relaxation and stress reduction
growth becoming	activities that improves knowledge and skills
physical belonging	home, neighborhood, community
social belonging	intimate others, family, friends, neighborhood and community
community belonging	adequate income, health and social services, recreational programs, community events and activities

4   Service Model for the Elderly

The Activities of Daily Living (ADLs) are a defined set of activities necessary for normal self-care. Six activities are defined by the Veteran Review Board [11]. Results in [12] suggest that the ADLs performed by elderly and the general population are similarly affected by need, enabling, and predisposing factors. From caregivers' perceptions, Roberto [1] presented assistances needed in personal and instrumental ADLs. This paper categorizes services needed by elderly into the following three groups:

Being-based elderly services are intended to help elderly to identify the help they need and the situation. These kinds of services keep both elderly people and their caregivers informed of issues and solutions for physical health (personal hygiene, nutrition, exercise, clothing, and general physical appearance), psychological health (mental and emotional), and spiritual health. **Becoming-based elderly services** seek to help elderly carry out purposeful activities such as domestic activities, and seeing to health or social needs. **Belonging-based elderly services** enable elderly people to connect with their families, friends, neighborhoods, or communities.

5   The Framework

Powered by context awareness and service computing, the framework, Pervasive Service Computing for the Elderly (PSC4E), defines an embedded, user-friendly computing and communication environment. This computer-enabled environment helps elderly users to easily access the above defined services, which currently must usually be physically delivered by caregivers. With wireless sensing devices embedded in the physical environment, PSC4E is available to deliver being-based services to help elderly people identify their health status. PSC4E provides timely transfer of information on people's health status to their caregivers, enabling real-time monitoring of activities and health conditions. PSC4E is also able to deliver becoming-based services, such as seeing a doctor or buying medicines. And PSC4E delivers belonging-based services to help elderly people at home to communicate with friends and doctors. The elderly can access PSC4E services via home tablets [46], smart phones, touch screens, or digital TVs. We propose a PSC4E framework (Figure 1) to pursue independent ageing through ubiquitously accommodating being-based, becoming-based, and belonging-based services. The four layers of the framework are presented next.

Context-Aware Middleware. Context is any information characterizing the situation of a task session, or interaction between a user and his/her service world. Context is categorized into five aspects, namely user context, peer context, process context, physical context, and service context [13][14]. A typical context-aware middleware has components of context sensing, context modeling, and context reasoning. Context sensing collects data from physical sensors measuring the elderly person's health condition, and his or her local environment. Context modeling abstracts description of sensing data. Context reasoning examines the contextual information and determines the elderly person's situation. Context Toolkit [15] and Context Fabric [16] are examples of general purpose context-aware middleware; CAMPH [17] and HYCARE [18] are context-aware middleware examples dedicated to healthcare.

Service Composition Middleware. Service composition describes a model of developing applications by integrating internet-accessible and discoverable loosely-coupled Web services [19]. A general purpose service composition middleware consists of components for composition planning, service discovery, service composition, and composition monitoring. Composition planning analyzes elderly persons' service requests, and initiates a work plan that composes the available services in the service repository to satisfy the service request. Service discovery matches services in the service repository against service requirements (input/output and QoS, etc.), and ranks them. Service composition establishes invocations and bindings among selected services, evaluates the plans, and identifies the best plan for the execution. The monitoring engine executes the plan and controls composition execution.

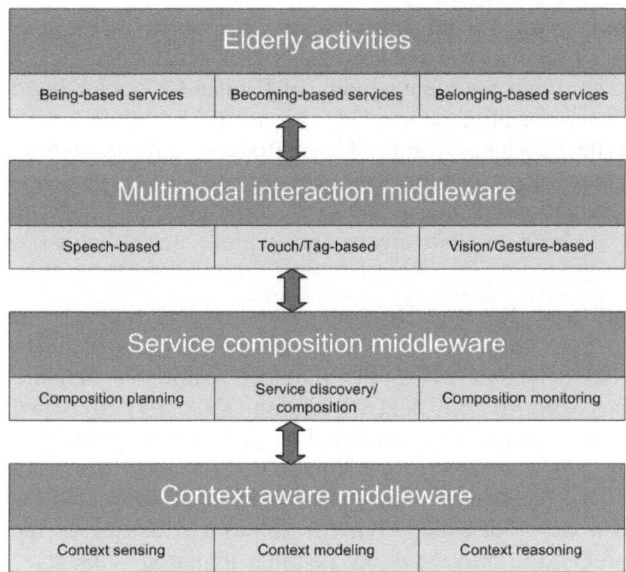

Fig. 1. The PSC4E Framework

Multimodal Interaction Middleware. As elderly people commonly have reduced abilities in areas such as vision, hearing and touch, we must provide them with multiple interactive interfaces. There are several different human computer interaction techniques which can help. PSC4E multimodal interface design [20] aims to adapt itself to the elderly person's needs using interactive visual, gesture, touch, speech, or tag-based interactions.

Elderly Services and Activities Layer. From the application point of view, the elderly often suffer from severe activity limitations, which may involve mobility, hearing, speaking, cognition, and social skills. Elderly service research focuses on systematically identifying basic needs for assisting elderly people's ADLs, and abstracting those needs as a service middleware of being-based services, becoming-based services, and belonging-based services that facilitates various agile healthcare application developments.

6   Related Studies

Assisting People with Movement Impairment. Movement impairment can make it difficult or impossible to use the hands, to walk, or move the trunk and neck [21]. Assistive devices that can compensate for movement impairment are such as canes, walkers, or wheelchairs. Recent advances in wheelchairs have produced "smart wheelchairs," which employ multimodal user interfaces with the user's senses of seeing, hearing, touch, taste, or smell [40–42][22][23] [24].

Assisting People with Visual Impairment. High-tech assistive products include video magnifiers, such as the pocket-sized pico, which gives an inverse white on black image [21]. There are many studies of Human-Computer Interfaces which can support interactions for blind people [25]. Alonso [26] presents a set of guidelines for blind user interface design. Evreinov [25] introduces a novel automated book reader as an assistive technology tool for blind persons. Challis [27] presents a system for the non-visual presentation of music notation. Albert [28] introduces a system that permits blind students to both create and explore mathematical graphics without assistance.

Assisting Deaf and Hard-of-Hearing. Hearing loss impacts on isolation and depression. To help with this, low tech assistive devices include vibrating alarm clocks and smoke detectors [21]. In the high tech realm, one example is development of smart phones with voice to text translation. Kakuta [29] created a prototype of VUTE, a communication aid system based on motion pictograms that can be used for hard-of-hearing people in emergency situations. Lozano [30] has studied techniques and algorithms for the detection and classification of household sounds. Ottaviano [31] presented a web tool called Gym2Learn, which focuses on metacognition and reading comprehension processes in hearing impaired students. Bumbalek [32] presented a web-based e-Scribe prototype for real-time speech transcription. Othman [33] proposed a web-based application to edit sports news in sign languages to keep deaf people informed of sports results.

Assisting People with Speech Impairment. Schultz [34] studied silent speech recognition based on Electromyography. Hamidi [35] developed a customizable speech recognition interface, CanSpeak, for the user. Gebert [36] demonstrated the conception and implementation of a language laboratory for speech reading.

Assisting People with Cognitive Problems. About 10% people over age 65 have cognitive impairments [21][4]. To cope with this, a special thematic session organized by Edler [37] aimed to study guidelines for accessible information to the World Wide Web. Bohman [38] examined the structure, navigation, language and the presentation of information on web sites in order to make internet accessible for people with reading problems. Matausch [39] presented a study on Easy-to-Read and its impacts on the support of people with specific learning difficulties.

Smart and Assistive Environments. Many studies concern smart and assistive environments. Morandell [40] organized a series of workshops on Ambient Assisted Living, in terms of ICT-based homecare and social interaction of elderly persons. Øystein [41] surveyed reports on the use of a GPS-based localization and tracking device for use in dementia care. Joan [42] developed the concept of a friendly and adapted robotized kitchen. Roel [43] presented the user-centered design of a medicine dispenser for persons suffering from Alzheimer's disease.

7   Conclusions and Future Work

ICT-based healthcare applications are evolving to improve the quality of life of the elderly. Current ICT-based applications [7] include mobile telemedicine; remote patient monitoring; location-based services; pervasive access to medical data; health-aware mobile devices; and lifestyle incentive management. There are several challenges to overcome in providing technological solutions in healthcare for the elderly [44]. PSC4E advances pervasive healthcare and incorporates emerging web services into healthcare service delivery. Taking advantages of context awareness and service composition, we regard PSC4E as a next generation technology targeting at an integrated platform for delivering personalized elderly healthcare, and supporting elderly people's ADLs through a simple unified user interface. In the study course of pervasive service computing, we have already implemented context-aware and service-oriented application prototypes for assisting campus activities, e.g., music recommendation and multimedia annotation [47]. Our plan is to implement prototypes to the elderly healthcare area based on our earlier work, to gain experience about the application, and verify the PSC4E framework. Future tasks in PSC4E are initially identified as follows:

Ontology-Based PSC4E Context Modeling. To facilitate elderly people's ADLs through personal service delivery, PSC4E needs to adapt to context changes and user configurations. Context modeling provides structures for capturing contextual information surrounding elderly persons. Context modeling is available for converting contextual information to a usable form through interpretation. Ontologies are widely accepted as instruments for the modeling of context information. This task explores ontology engineering and context modeling in information management for PSC4E.

PSC4E Activity Modeling. PSC4E targets delivering services for facilitating elderly user's ADLs at a high level. This gives rise to PSC4E activity modeling. PSC4E aims to present a representation mechanism for rules, conditions, constraints, controls, and data dependencies in elderly people's ADLs.

PSC4E in Cloud Computing. Cloud computing describes a model of sharing a pool of configurable computing resources in a rapid-provisioning, minimal management manner. PSC4E in Cloud Computing aims to study the application of Cloud Computing in delivery of elderly services and health data.

Acknowledgements. This work was financially supported by the Ubiquitous Computing and Diversity of Communication (MOTIVE) program of the Academy of Finland and carried out during the first author's visiting research hosted by Prof. Hans-Arno Jacobsen from Middleware Research Group at University of Toronto.

References

[1]   Roberto, K.A.: The Elderly Caregiver: Caring for Adults with Developmental Disabilities. SAGE, Newbury (1993)
[2]   Rowe, J.W., Kahn, R.L.: Human Aging: Usual and Successful. Science 237, 143–149 (1987)
[3]   Strawbridge, W.J., Wallhagen, M.I., Cohen, R.D.: Successful Aging and Well-being: Self-rated Compared with Rowe and Kahn. The Gerontologist 42, 727–733 (2002)

[4]   Davenport, R.D.: Robotics. In: Mann, W.C. (ed.) Smart Technology for Aging, Disability, and Independence: The State of the Science, pp. 67–110. John Wiley & Sons, Inc., Hoboken (2005)

[5]   Kidd, C.D., Orr, R., Abowd, G.D., Atkeson, C.G., Macintyre, I.A.B., Mynatt, E., Starner, T.E., Newstetter, W.: The Aware Home: A Living Laboratory for Ubiquitous Computing Research. In: Proceedings of the Second International Workshop on Cooperative Buildings, Integrating Information, Organization, and Architecture, pp. 191–198 (1999)

[6]   Dowdall, A., Perry, M.: The Millennium Home: Domestic Technology to Support Independent-Living Older People. In: Proceedings of the 1st Equator IRC Workshop, pp. 1–15 (2001)

[7]   Stanford, V.: Using Pervasive Computing to Deliver Elder Care. IEEE Pervasive Computing 1, 10–13 (2002)

[8]   United Nations: World Population Ageing (2009), http://www.un.org/esa/population/publications/WPA2009/ WPA2009_WorkingPaper.pdf (accessed by March 9, 2010)

[9]   Schalock, R.L.: Quality of Life for People with Intellectual and Other Developmental Disabilities: Applications Across Individuals, Organizations, Communities, and Systems. American Association on Intellectual and Developmental Disabilities, Washington, DC (2007)

[10] Dennis, R., Browna, I., Renwicka, R., Rootmana, I.: Assessing the Quality of Life of Persons with Developmental Disabilities: Description of a New Model, Measuring Instruments, and Initial Findings. International J. of Disability, Development and Education 43, 25–42 (1996)

[11] Veteran Review Board. Activities of Daily Living, http://www.vrb.gov.au/pubs/garp-chapter16.pdf (accessed by March 9, 2010)

[12] Coulton, C., Frost, A.K.: Use of Social and Health Services by the Elderly. J of Health and Social Behavior 23, 330–339 (1982)

[13] Zhou, J., Gilman, E., Palola, J., Riekki, J., Ylianttila, M., Sun, J.: Context-Aware Pervasive Service Composition and Its Implementation. Personal and Ubiquitous Computing 15, 291–303 (2011)

[14] Zhou, J., Riekki, J.: Context-Aware Pervasive Service Composition. In: Proceedings of International Conference on Intelligent Systems, Modeling and Simulation, pp. 437–442 (2010)

[15] Salber, D., Dey, D., Abowd, A.K., G.D.: The Context Toolkit: Aiding the Development of Context-Enabled Applications. In: Proceedings of the SIGCHI Conference on Human Factors in Computing Systems: The CHI is the Limit, pp. 434–441 (1999)

[16] Hong, J.I.: The Context Fabric: An Infrastructure for Context-Aware Computing. In: Proceedings of CHI 2002 Extended Abstracts on Human Factors in Computing Systems, pp. 554–555 (2002)

[17] Hung, K.P., Tao, G., Wenwei, X., Palmes, P.P., Jian, Z., Wen, L.N., Chee, W.T., Weng, T., Nguyen, H.C.: Context-Aware Middleware for Pervasive Elderly Homecare. IEEE J. on Selected Areas in Communications 27, 510–524 (2009)

[18] Du, K., Zhang, D., Zhou, X., Mokhtari, M., Hariz, M., Qin, W.: HYCARE: A Hybrid Context-Aware Reminding Framework for Elders with Mild Dementia. In: Helal, S., Mitra, S., Wong, J., Chang, C.K., Mokhtari, M. (eds.) ICOST 2008. LNCS, vol. 5120, pp. 9–17. Springer, Heidelberg (2008)

[19] Zhou, J., Gilman, E., Riekki, J., Rautiainen, M., Ylianttila, M.: Ontology-Driven Pervasive Service Composition for Everyday Life. In: Margaria, T., Steffen, B. (eds.) ISoLA 2010. LNCS, vol. 6415, pp. 375–389. Springer, Heidelberg (2010)

[20] Zhou, J., Junzhao, S., Athukorala, K., Wijekoon, D.: Pervasive Social Computing: Augmenting Five Facets of Human Intelligence. In: Proceedings of Ubiquitous Intelligence & Computing and 7th International Conference on Autonomic & Trusted Computing (UIC/ATC), pp. 1–6. Springer, Heidelberg (2010)

[21] Mann, W.C.: Aging, Disability and Independence: Trends and Perspectives. In: Mann, W. (ed.) Smart Technology for Aging, Disability, and Independence: The State of the Science. John Wiley & Sons, Inc., Hoboken (2005)

[22] Kim, H., Ryu, D.: Smart Wheelchair Based on Ultrasonic Positioning System. In: Miesenberger, K., Klaus, J., Zagler, W.L., Karshmer, A.I. (eds.) ICCHP 2006. LNCS, vol. 4061, pp. 1014–1020. Springer, Heidelberg (2006)

[23] Mayer, P., Panek, P., Edelmayer, G., Nuttin, M., Zagler, W.L.: Scenarios of Use for a Modular Robotic Mobility Enhancement System for Profoundly Disabled Children in an Educational and Institutional Care Environment. In: Miesenberger, K., Klaus, J., Zagler, W.L., Karshmer, A.I. (eds.) ICCHP 2006. LNCS, vol. 4061, pp. 1021–1028. Springer, Heidelberg (2006)

[24] Simpson, R.C.: Smart Wheelchairs: A Literature Review. J. Rehabil. Res. Dev. 42(4), 423–436 (2005)

[25] Evreinov, G.: Blind and Visually Impaired People: Human Computer Interface. In: Miesenberger, K., Klaus, J., Zagler, W.L., Karshmer, A.I. (eds.) ICCHP 2006. LNCS, vol. 4061, pp. 1029–1030. Springer, Heidelberg (2006)

[26] Alonso, F., Fuertes, J., González, Á., Martínez, L.: A Framework for Blind User Interfacing. In: Miesenberger, K., Klaus, J., Zagler, W.L., Karshmer, A.I. (eds.) ICCHP 2006. LNCS, vol. 4061, pp. 1031–1038. Springer, Heidelberg (2006)

[27] Challis, B.P.: Accessing Music Notation Through Touch and Speech. In: Miesenberger, K., Klaus, J., Zagler, W.L., Karshmer, A.I. (eds.) ICCHP 2006. LNCS, vol. 4061, pp. 1110–1117. Springer, Heidelberg (2006)

[28] Albert, P.: Math Class: An Application for Dynamic Tactile Graphics. In: Miesenberger, K., Klaus, J., Zagler, W.L., Karshmer, A.I. (eds.) ICCHP 2006. LNCS, vol. 4061, pp. 1118–1121. Springer, Heidelberg (2006)

[29] Kakuta, M., Nakazono, K., Nagashima, Y., Hosono, N.: Development of Universal Communication Aid for Emergency Using Motion Pictogram. In: Miesenberger, K., Klaus, J., Zagler, W., Karshmer, A. (eds.) ICCHP 2010. LNCS, vol. 6179, pp. 308–311. Springer, Heidelberg (2010)

[30] Lozano, H., Hernáez, I., Picón, A., Camarena, J., Navas, E.: Audio Classification Techniques in Home Environments for Elderly/Dependant People. In: Miesenberger, K., Klaus, J., Zagler, W., Karshmer, A. (eds.) ICCHP 2010. LNCS, vol. 6179, pp. 320–323. Springer, Heidelberg (2010)

[31] Ottaviano, S., Merlo, G., Chifari, A., Chiazzese, G., Seta, L., Allegra, M., Samperi, V.: The Deaf and Online Comprehension Texts: How Can Technology Help? In: Miesenberger, K., Klaus, J., Zagler, W., Karshmer, A. (eds.) ICCHP 2010. LNCS, vol. 6180, pp. 144–151. Springer, Heidelberg (2010)

[32] Bumbalek, Z., Zelenka, J., Kencl, L.: E-Scribe: Ubiquitous Real-Time Speech Transcription for the Hearing-Impaired. In: Miesenberger, K., Klaus, J., Zagler, W., Karshmer, A. (eds.) ICCHP 2010. LNCS, vol. 6180, pp. 160–168. Springer, Heidelberg (2010)

[33] Othman, A., El Ghoul, O., Jemni, M.: SportSign: A Service to Make Sports News Accessible to Deaf Persons in Sign Languages. In: Miesenberger, K., Klaus, J., Zagler, W., Karshmer, A. (eds.) ICCHP 2010. LNCS, vol. 6180, pp. 169–176. Springer, Heidelberg (2010)

[34] Weber, G.: ICCHP Keynote: Recognizing Silent and Weak Speech Based on Electromyography. In: Miesenberger, K., Klaus, J., Zagler, W., Karshmer, A. (eds.) ICCHP 2010. LNCS, vol. 6180, pp. 431–438. Springer, Heidelberg (2010)

[35] Hamidi, F., Baljko, M., Livingston, N., Spalteholz, L.: CanSpeak: a Customizable Speech Interface for People with Dysarthric Speech. In: Miesenberger, K., Klaus, J., Zagler, W., Karshmer, A. (eds.) ICCHP 2010. LNCS, vol. 6179, pp. 605–612. Springer, Heidelberg (2010)

[36] Gebert, H., Bothe, H.-H.: LIPPS—A Virtual Teacher for Speechreading Based on a Dialog-Controlled Talking-Head. In: Miesenberger, K., Klaus, J., Zagler, W., Karshmer, A. (eds.) ICCHP 2010. LNCS, vol. 6179, pp. 621–629. Springer, Heidelberg (2010)

[37] Edler, C., Peböck, B.: Easy-to-Web: Introduction to the Special Thematic Session. In: Miesenberger, K., Klaus, J., Zagler, W., Karshmer, A. (eds.) ICCHP 2010. LNCS, vol. 6179, pp. 630–633. Springer, Heidelberg (2010)

[38] Bohman, U.: The Need for Easy-to-Read Information on Web Sites. In: Miesenberger, K., Klaus, J., Zagler, W., Karshmer, A. (eds.) ICCHP 2010. LNCS, vol. 6179, pp. 634–640. Springer, Heidelberg (2010)

[39] Matausch, K., Peböck, B.: EasyWeb—A Study How People with Specific Learning Difficulties Can Be Supported on Using the Internet. In: Miesenberger, K., Klaus, J., Zagler, W., Karshmer, A. (eds.) ICCHP 2010. LNCS, vol. 6179, pp. 641–648. Springer, Heidelberg (2010)

[40] Morandell, M., Fugger, E.: Results of a Workshop Series on Ambient Assisted Living. In: Miesenberger, K., Klaus, J., Zagler, W., Karshmer, A. (eds.) ICCHP 2010. LNCS, vol. 6179, pp. 288–291. Springer, Heidelberg (2010)

[41] Dale, Ø.: Usability and Usefulness of GPS Based Localization Technology Used in Dementia Care. In: Miesenberger, K., Klaus, J., Zagler, W., Karshmer, A. (eds.) ICCHP 2010. LNCS, vol. 6179, pp. 300–307. Springer, Heidelberg (2010)

[42] Aranda, J., Vinagre, M., Martín, E.X., Casamitjana, M., Casals, A.: Friendly Human-Machine Interaction in an Adapted Robotized Kitchen. In: Miesenberger, K., Klaus, J., Zagler, W., Karshmer, A. (eds.) ICCHP 2010. LNCS, vol. 6179, pp. 312–319. Springer, Heidelberg (2010)

[43] de Beer, R., Keijers, R., Shahid, S., Al Mahmud, A., Mubin, O.: PMD: Designing a Portable Medicine Dispenser for Persons Suffering from Alzheimer's Disease. In: Miesenberger, K., Klaus, J., Zagler, W., Karshmer, A. (eds.) ICCHP 2010. LNCS, vol. 6179, pp. 332–335. Springer, Heidelberg (2010)

[44] Varshney, U.: Pervasive Healthcare. Computer 36, 138–140 (2003)

[45] National Institutes of Health, Research Plan for the National Center for Medical Rehabilitation Research (March 1993),
http://www.nichd.nih.gov/publications/pubs/upload/plan.pdf
(accessed by March 9, 2011)

[46] Archos 7. Home Tablet (2011), http://www.archos.com/ (accessed by March 9, 2011)

[47] Zhou, J., Riekki, J., Ylianttila, M., Zhou, J., Tang, F., Guo, M.: State of the art on Pervasive Service Computing. In: Proc. International Workshop on Ubiquitous Healthcare and Welfare Services and Supporting Technologies, pp. 1–6 (2010)

[48] e-Inclusion, e-Inclusion (2011),
http://ec.europa.eu/information_society/activities/
einclusion/index_en.htm (accessed by March 9, 2011)

[49] AAL, Ambient Assisted Living Joint Programme (2011),
http://www.aal-europe.eu/ (accessed by March 9, 2011)

Alert Calls in Remote Health:
Cultural Adaptation and Usability Inspection for China

Timo Korhonen[1], Xirui Wang[1], Shuo Liu[1], Christos Karaiskos[1], and Yuping Zhao[2]

[1] Dept. of Communications and Networking, Aalto University, Espoo, Finland
`firstname.lastname@tkk.fi`
[2] Satellite & Wireless Communication Laboratory,
Peking University, China
`yuping.zhao@pku.edu.cn`

Abstract. In this paper we inspect remote health care, and especially alert call concept and usability design for Chinese Chronic Obstructive Pulmonary Disease (COPD) patients. Generally, remote health care can facilitate cost efficient and improved treatment and follow-up of various illnesses. For service providers it can offer expanded service palette, enable easier access of medical information and support new business models. However, when the service works in a multi-cultural environment, related cultural factors need also be considered in service design that we investigate in this paper where we suggest a systematic methodology. Also, respective usability evaluation is addressed.

Keywords: Elderly care, usability, service localization, COPD, cultural service adaptation.

1   Introduction

By the year of 2050, the world will count 2 billion people over the age of 60. As forChina, the number of citizens aged over 50 grows from 22% to 29% [1]. Urbanization, aging, and changes in globalized lifestyle result more chronic illnesses and mental distress. Diabetes, cardiovascular diseases, depression and cancers are increasing especially amongst elderly. In this study, we focus particularly on Chronic Obstructive Pulmonary Disease (COPD), which is a life-threatening, progressive lung disease blocking airflow into lungs, and causing short of breath.

There are several factors bringing serious challenges to health care and wellbeing sector. These include especially increasing costs of medical technology, medication, and labor. This reflects, for instance, in shortage of beds and nursing houses. Additionally, realization of consumerism is growing significantly in the field of health care. By consumerism we refer to the general trend that patients are demanding more information and more frequent communication with caregivers, and more diversity in services. Also, patients' responsibility of taking care of themselves is highlighted.

Therefore, well being technologies and services are also developing rapidly. In order to satisfy the consumers, patient-centric care is required, with patients and their

M. Rautiainen et al. (Eds.): GPC 2011 Workshops, LNCS 7096, pp. 83–93, 2012.

service providers sharing personalized and contextual health information and treatment access [2].

One of the enabling technologies is mobile communications. There were 786.50 million subscribers of mobile communication services in China by the end of April 2010, growing by 1.24% monthly and by 15.87% yearly [3]. Mobile communications offers a rapidly developing, pervasive platform for implementing remote health care. This supports the following advantages of remote health care over conventional heath care: Firstly, it is easier for elders to access medical information, daily life services, and have even cognitive exercises via intelligent phones [4]. Secondly, for health service providers, remote health care facilitates information exchange and delivery, social and emotional support. Moreover, as the telephony services have become wireless, they are thus also more ubiquitous, that can greatly improve safety and security, for instance by providing true 24/7 full-duplex accessibility.

Our paper is organized as follows: In Section 2, the significance of studying COPD in China is illustrated. Section 3 discusses how alert calls can reduce costs for patients and governments. Section 4 focuses on general cultural service transfer theory of services and Section 5 to user centered design for elderly. Sections 6 and 7 discuss medical alert calls and the inspected COPD – case, respectively. Section 8 analyzes the targeted user-centered design issues and finally cultural service concept transfer is addressed in Section 9. Paper is ended with conclusions in Section 10.

2   COPD in China

COPD is caused by breathing of noxious particles or gases, such as cigarette smoking and second-hand smoke, air pollution, and other occupational pollutants. Although COPD is considered a lifestyle disease which can be prevented by adoption of a healthy lifestyle, it is non-reversible condition. Around 3 million people die in COPD annually. In China, COPD ranks number one among the burdens of diseases. It is the 2nd leading cause of death, over one million people die and five million people are disabled due to COPD annually [5].

Smoking is the major cause of COPD in China. There are 320 million smokers, which makes up to 1/3 of the smokers worldwide [6]. Unlike in other countries, there are 38.6% of non-smokers suffering COPD in China, of which 44.6% suffers of COPD that is caused of burning biomass materials for cooking [7]. Passive smoking also contributes to COPD prevalence in non-smokers; research among Chinese men and women aged over 50 has shown that people experiencing high levels of passive smoking, greater or equal to 40 hours per week, are 48% more likely to develop COPD [8]. Currently, there are 25 million people in China having COPD, which costs for the society are high in healthcare expenditures, and in medical resource [9]. For instance, it is estimated that 36% of COPD patients miss directly 17 working days per year due to COPD attacks. 17% of COPD patients' family members are absent from their work, making in average 14 days per year for the reason that they need to take care of the COPD patients. This naturally lowers societal productivity and economic growth too [10]. Therefore, China must now face the importance of COPD, and try to actively search solutions to the worsening situation.

3   Some Cost Considerations

Chinese Labour Insurance Regulations was issued by Government Administration Council by the year 1951; the retirement age for male is 60, and 50 for female. Although, several changes have been made to modify the retirement age (for instance some occupations have a significantly lower retirement age), the early retirement age still brings a significant pressure onto the society, especially in healthcare. Most people over 60 have a low productivity and their life dependents on governmental pension [11]. They suffer usually various illnesses that the chronic diseases tend to be also costly requiring intense, long-term treatment. However, most medical costs can be reimbursed by the governmental healthcare insurance also in China [12]. Some costs for COPD are estimated in Table 1 based on interviews we conducted in China in 2010 [13]. The less elderly enter medical treatments or visit hospitals, the more society funds are saved. Alert calls can suppress/milder illnesses attacks and reduce hospital visits and durations. Thus patients and society are saving both money and time.

In this research we focus on COPD remote alert calls that were first piloted in Cornwall, UK [14]. The system applied automated telephone calls to alert people with COPD to periods when the Met Office COPD Health Forecast indicated that their risk of illness was 'elevated', either as a result of high risk weather (such as cold), high levels of respiratory infections or both. The practices that used the service reduced COPD hospital admission rates by 52% when compared to the previous year. This reduction equates to a potential saving of up to GBP 300,000 in each winter. Thus the benefits of COPD alert calls are clear in this case. However, customer satisfaction and service efficiency are also function of overall service design and user interface detailing. Also, we are interested to understand, how the UK COPD alert call realization could be localized for China that we next inspect.

Table 1. Approximating COPD costs in Shandong Provincial Hospital, China, 2010 [12]

Condition	Mild	Average	Serious / surgery
Frequency	1 – 2 times per year	4 – 10 times / year	more than 10 times/ year
Total Costs	1650 RMB	25500 RMB	40800 RMB
Other Costs	150 RMB	500 RMB	800 RMB
Surgery	No	No	15000 RMB
Hospitalization period	No	1-3 months	1-5 months
Hospitalization	No	25000 RMB	25000 RMB
Medication & Injection	1500 RMB		

4   Cultural Service Adaptation

In transformation of services between cultures, characteristics of both cultures need to be addressed and the actual service needs to be parameterized (Fig. 1b). To start with, cultural characterization can be based on Hofstede's cultural dimensioning that divides the cultural effects into several sub-properties [17]. These include Power Distance (PDI), Avoidance of Uncertainties (UAI), Masculinity Index (MAS), Collectivism/Individualism (IDV), and Long-term/Short-term orientation (LTO). Estimates of these parameters are shown in Fig. 1a for China and Finland.

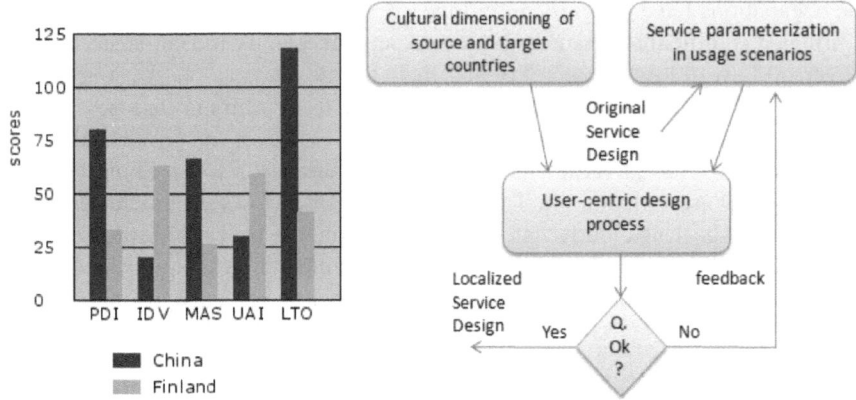

Fig. 1. a) Geert Hofstede's cultural dimensions for China and Finland [18]. PDI: (Chi 80/Fin 33), IDV: (Chi 20/Fin 63), MAS: (Chi 66/Fin 26), UAI: (Chi30/Fin 59), LTO: (Chi 118/Fin 41) 1b) Cultural service adaption process. Design quality control (indicated by Q. in the diagram) is based on monitoring design quality indicators or cultural metrics. These can be for instance attributes in menus/navigation, controls, conceptual models or appear in overall fitness for usage.

Also, individuals can be culturally classified following Hofstede's cultural dimensioning, or some other classification [19]. Generally, cultural orientation of humans is a result of personal and society related factors. Therefore, cultural service adaptation should consider the target group users and society simultaneously. Culture reflects clearly in language and in thinking styles in general, that carry a historical framework. For further information, see for instance Nisbett, who has addressed especially thinking in the East and the West [20]. For cultural adaption of services, also service concept needs to be first well-defined. For this, service concept should be functionally and culturally analyzed using some relevant usage scenarios [21]. This aims to identification and understanding of functions of culture related factors in the service, which can then be used to localize the service design for the particular target country.

Design of user interface needs usually to be updated in cultural service transfer. This is inspected for instance by Marcus [22]. Required adjustments stipulate artistic, technical and societal expertise in understanding of culture, services and users in both source and target countries. Also, cross-disciplinary, multi-cultural focus groups should be used for evaluations in the various phases of the user centric design process intermediate outputs and piloting. Resulting data and findings should then be injected back to the service concept design, for instance by using adjustable mock-ups [23]. Mock-ups are jointly tuned in the design process by professional service designers and intended users.

5   User-Centered Design for Elderly

User-centric design process aims to realize usable products and services. Generally, usability refers to effectiveness, efficiency, and satisfaction by which the targeted users can achieve some, well-defined goals within a specified usage scenario. Scenario elements are scenes, actors, objective, plans, evaluations, acts and happenings [24], [25]. By definition, effectiveness indicates accuracy and completeness that the users accomplish the goals. Efficiency is defined as the relation between the effectiveness and the resources used in achieving goals [26]. In the focus of this study, user scenario describes the remote COPD alert call service applying numerical keypad and auditive interface.

Contemporary usability evaluation methodologies can be classified into three categories [26][27]: Usability testing, usability inspection, and usability inquiry. For usability testing, service can be evaluated with the actual users and/or experts. The objective is to find out how well practical usability design (traditionally especially user interface) supports accessing the service concept features.

For the aged population, accessibility problems, lack of knowledge and poor earlier user experience are a major complication in adaptation of almost any ICT - services.

Physical and mental capabilities of elders are often reduced. Elderly prefer traditionally face-to-face communication and do not easily rely on technology-mediated services. Elderly can own a low computer literacy and confidence and some higher ethical concerns in privacy, autonomy, integrity, dignity, and reliability [28]. However, there is now a growing population in older ages that already has more experience in using developed ICT - services. Therefore internet-based social media tools, such as Facebook, or even special, elderly tailored social portals have started to appear and gain popularity [29]. Furthermore, usage of mobile phone is becoming increasingly common among elders, due to the feeling of security of being ubiquitously reachable. This has triggered mobile companies to focus on usability concepts accustomed to elderly needs; large-size screens for better view, large-size keypads for better reach, vibration and blinking lights for better hearing [30]. In summary, successful service design for elderly should always carefully consider all of these challenges.

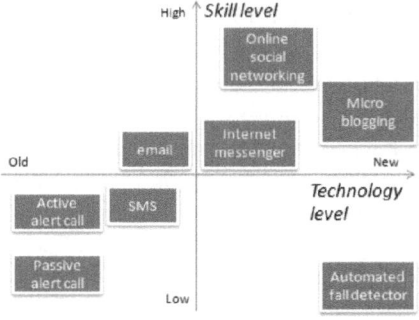

Fig. 2. Comparing remote health alert service access in terms of technologic development timeline and required usage skill

6   Medical Alert Calls

Let us now focus on alert call services that can be divided to start with, into passiveand active calls and they can apply wired or mobile terminals. In the active calls, user can initiate a predefined calling sequence [31][32] and in the passive calls, 24/7 supervising alert center makes the call. Active initiation can be triggered by pressing a panic button, e.g., on a pendant, bracelet, or in some other, custom-designed phone-attached service terminal [33]. After pressing the button, alarm is passed to alert center. Then the center alerts ambulances and/or forwards the alert to some other required authorities, as firemen or police. However, earlier studies indicate that the alert center can add a significant delay while answering the call, looking up the medical records, and analyzing the call. In order to reduce this delay, some service providers connect subscriber directly to a certain, close-proximity help providing party, as neighbors or relatives [31]. However, generally active alert calls can be very effective in elderly (around and above 65 years) falling incidents: After a fall or other emergency, 90% of people who get help within one hour will continue independent living, but after 12 hours without help only 10% of people will continue to live at home [36]. Elderly falls account for one-third of all non-fatal injuries and hospitalizations in US [37]. Injuries caused by falling were the main reason for fatal accidents in Finland, reaching 64.4% among other accident types, such as poisoning by alcohol or transport accidents in the year 2009 [34].

Alert calls can also be divided with respect of network access/user interface, suchas those using short message services (SMS) [35] or emails [12] (Fig. 2). New Internet-based tools, like micro-blogging [15], instant messaging, video chat, onlinesocial networks, and cloud services are changing the ways the alerts are delivered [16]. Relating service ecosystems are also developing. Medical alert calls form aninteresting group in the wide palette of remote health care services. They can also have a very limited number of features if realized by fixed line, conventional keypadphones. This sets stringent requirements for service and user interface design.

In this paper, we here on focus on passive medical alert calls. In contrast to activealert calls, system initiates the passive calls. The initiation can be time- or event-triggered [38].

7   Medical Alert Call for COPD – Service Functionalities

The interactive, passive, COPD pilot we focus here [14], asked patients two evidence based questions about their condition to which they answer simply 'yes' or 'no' by selecting the respective keypad number that is then relayed to the doctor or nurse. Five calls were made to each patient during the winter, in response to the prevailing COPD conditions. Service has the following functionalities: 1. Service Introduction: This gives some brief information about the alert call service and target illness. 2. User Verification: System verifies whether the intended patient has been reached. If the verification fails, system informs the person the intention of this alert call and schedules another date to call. 3. Alert Message: User exchanges the alert messages (e.g., informs of the possible condition deterioration, running out of medicines, reminds of doctor appointment...). 4. Questions: There is a set of questions for the patients to confirm and check whether they are prepared for the problems illustrated in the alert messages. 5. Good-bye message: System schedules time for the next call and informs the user.

8   Analyzing User-Centric Design

Let us now inspect usability aspects of the targeted service where we have applied cognitive walkthrough and heuristic evaluation. The results are discussed as follows:

First the identified usability problem is highlighted, then the implications from the problem are discussed, and in the end, design improvements for the particular problems are suggested.

A.   Lack of accelerators or skip-functions
The introduction of the service provider, alert call service and the illness takes more than 30 second for every call. This information is, no doubt, beneficial for novice user. Nonetheless, after using the service in cognitive walkthrough, this piece of information became soon frustrating. Therefore, we would argue that for experienced users, the introductory part can be frustrating only. An accelerator could be used to speed up the interactions between the system and the experienced users. Basic implementation of accelerator could function as a fast-forward button in some conventional media player. Also, a skip-functionality could be applied. Advanced implementation could even allow users to tailor their frequent actions for future.

B.   Question repetition
In the question round, the alert call system is designed such as in case of no-response for 15 seconds, the automatic question repetition is triggered. Moreover, this is the only way to replay the question. This indicates lack of user control, low flexibility and user interface inefficiency. Hence, a dedicated function for repeating question dialogs or any statements should be added, for example, by pressing an assigned keypad entry. Repetition function could be enabled throughout the whole alert call service. Whenever the user fails to keep in pace with the system, they could trigger the repetition immediately. This functionality would be announced in service introduction - phase. By adding this functionality users would get some sense of control, avoid frustration and save time. The benefits would become still greater with long and complex statements or questions.

C.   Error Prevention and User Control
Some usability problems appeared in the question rounds as well. Every time when the user committed an action by pressing the assigned keypad entry, the system responded by repeating user's choice and then proceeding to the next question. We found out in cognitive walkthrough that in case of incorrect choice (keying in a wrong number), there was no way for take back except hanging the phone and then waiting for the next call to be initiated by the alarm center. Voice / keypad – only controlled

alert calls are challenging and error control can clearly be a problem. This is even more prominent with elderly having more often hearing deficiencies. Hence, undo or revocation functions could be implemented. However, this functionality (as also other suggested alterations) should be carefully tested for not to obscure general user interface clarity.

D. Learnability
The service has a lengthy flow diagram. There is a question how easy is it for elders to follow through this automated audio set of multiple steps? Elders do often have a limited attention volume. With complex and lengthy flow diagram, part of information is easily misunderstood or left unreachable.

E. Language and Personalization
In voice-based services, language as such requires a special attention. In order to find out language effects a throughout usability study would be in place also for this service. Especially, one should pay attention if the language is "senior-friendly" with respect of articulation, vocabulary, clarity, pitch, tone, spacing of sentences, and words.

9   Transforming the Service from Finland to China

All the five cultural dimensions discussed earlier can have more or less implications in particular services adaptation. Based on native Chinese analyzers authoring this paper, Power Distance, Individualism and Uncertainty Avoidance have a more significant impact when localizing the target service from Finland to China. The other two dimensions, Long-term Orientation and Masculinity can have some impacts too, but we could not clearly identify their effect in this study. Note anyhow that their deviation between Finland and China is large (MAS: Chi 66/Fin 26, LTO: Chi 118/Fin 41) (Fig. 1a). Let us therefore now focus on the other three cultural dimensions.

Finland, as the originator of the inspected remote alert call service, is characterize as an individualistic society with some extremely low Power Distance (Chi 8o/Fin 33) and moderate Uncertainty Avoidance index (Chi 30/Fin 49). China, as the destination of service transformation under study, can be described as a strong, collectivistic country (Individualism index: Chi 20 /Fin 63) embracing uncertainty some what better than Finns and keeping a significantly larger distances in societal hierarchies.

China ranks lower than any other Asian country in Individualism. In a collective society, people foster stronger relationships by taking more responsibility of fellow group members. Therefore Chinese elderly are willing to acknowledge own incapability and expect strong support from their relatives. For service design this implicates that there should be enhanced focus to offer good connections between elderly, their families and other friend, instead of one-dimensionally supporting their independence. Additionally, comparing to the western elderly who foster strong individualism, Chinese elders are also reluctant in decision-making. This indicates that requesting critical judgments and/or answers in queries through out the investigated service does not feel polite or even functional with Chinese elderly.

China has the highest Power Distance ranking of 80 compared to the other Far East Asian countries' having average of 60, and the world average of 55. This is an elementary part of cultural heritage in China. For the health care services, it indicates that the Chinese patients are more obedient to doctors and supporting system, which are considered to be in a higher power position. Therefore, they are expecting decisive, clear and command-like instructions in health services and treatments.

The Uncertainty Avoidance Index for China is quite low, in overall ranking of countries, 30 compared to Finland 59. This can be related to the complexity of user interface. High Uncertainty Avoidance countries prefer restricted options and simple controls, while with low Uncertainty Avoidance index, one prefers multiple options and complex controls.

10   Conclusions

Throughout our study, alert calls are seen to be clearly applicable and beneficial in remote health care of elderly. COPD alert calls can reduce number of unnecessary clinic visits and improve care quality in supervising medication intake and supplies. Medical alert calls carry also some potential societal benefits. For the patients, they can support more independent living and getting to be more aware of their sickness.

Alert calls are cheap and efficient way to improve quality of life and to cut treatment costs.

Based on this research, in remote alert calls menu construction (service flow chart), realization of help functions and linguistic style in general can be problematic. Elderly as the targeted user group sets further requirements in the service clarity. Based on our findings, usable cultural transfer of the inspected alert call service would likely require adjustment in all of these components.

At the moment, remote alert calls are applied in a very limited area. We believe that also other chronic illnesses, e.g., diabetes or hypertension, could greatly benefit of alert calls that we plan to extent our research too.

Acknowledgments. This research is supported by the Academy of Finland under grant no 129446.

References

1. Orr, G.R.: The Aging of China. McKinsey Quarterly (2004)
2. Simons, D.P.: Consumer Electronics: Opportunities in Remote and Home Healthcare. Philips Research
3. Ministry of Industry and Information Technology of the People's Republic of China, http://www.miit.gov.cn (accessed July 8, 2010)
4. Davis, R.N., Massman, P.J., Doody, R.S.: Cognitive Intervention in Alzheimer Disease: A Randomized Placebo-Controlled Study. Alzheimer Disease and Associated Disorders 15(1), 1–9

5. The Top 10 Causes of Death, World Health Organization, `http://www.who.int/mediacentre/factsheets/fs310/en/index.html` (accessed November 6, 2010)
6. Report on Chronic Disease in China: Ministry of Health of the People's Republic of China, Chinese Center for Disease Control and Prevention (May 2006)
7. Zhang, H., Cai, B.: The Impact of Tobacco on Lung Health in China. Respirology 8, 17–21 (2003), doi:10.1046/j.1440-1843.2003.00433.x
8. Passive Smoking Could Cause 1.9 Million Excess Deaths from COPD in China, `http://www.sciencedaily.com/releases/2007/08/070831203607.htm`
9. He, Q.: Chinese patients with chronic obstructive pulmonary disease status of study results. China Medical Tribune 9(33), 5 (2007)
10. Zhou, Y., Wang, C., Yao, W., Chen, P., Kang, J., Huang, S., Chen, B., Wang, C., Ni, D., Wang, X., Wang, D., Liu, S., Lu, J., Zheng, J., Zhong, N., Ran, P.: COPD in Chinese nonsmokers. European Respiratory Journal 33(3), 509–518 (2009)
11. Shao, G., Zhai, X.: Population Aging Challenges the Chinese Current Rule of Retirement Age (October 18, 2009), `http://www.csscipaper.com`
12. Baker, L., Wagner, T.H., Singer, S., Bundorf, M.K.: Use of the Internet and E-mail for Health Care Information. JAMA 289, 2400–2406 (2003)
13. Wang, M.: Interview, COPD in Shandong Province, Respiratory Department, Shandong Provincial Hospital, Shandong, China (September 15, 2010)
14. Sachon, P., Laing-Morten, T., Marno, P.: Pilot of an Automated Direct-to-Patient Health Forecasting System in Cornwall, South West England, for people with Chronic Obstructive Pulmonary Disease. In: EMS7/ECAM8 Abstracts EMS2007-A-00718, 7th EMS Annual Meeting/8th ECAM, vol. 4 (2007)
15. NEED Help!: Biker's Twitter followers call for ambulance, `http://www.usatoday.com/news/health/2010-08-03-twitterrescue03_st_N.htm` (accessed August 15, 2010)
16. Hawn, C.: Take Two Aspirin And Tweet Me In The Morning:How Twitter, Facebook, And Other Social Media Are Reshaping Health Care. Health Affairs 28(2), 361–368 (2009)
17. Hofstede, G.: Cultures and Organizations: Software of the Mind Intercultural Cooperation and its Importance for Survival. Harper- Collins Publishers, London (1994); ISBN: 0 00 637740 8
18. Geert Hofstede^{TM} Cultural Dimensions, `http://geert-hofstede.com/hofstede_dimensions.php?culture1=18&culture2=32#compare` (accessed March 15, 2011)
19. Schwartz, S.H.: A Theory of Cultural Values and Some Implications for Work. Applied Psychology: An International Review 48(1), 23–47 (1999)
20. Nisbett, R.: The Geography of Thought: How Asians and Westerners Think Differently and Why. The Free Press, USA (2003); ISBN: 0-7432-1646-6, Nisbett, M., Chang, J., Oxford University Press
21. Rosson, M.B., Carroll, J.M.: Usability Engineering, Scenario-Based Development of Human-Computer Interaction. Morgan Kaufmann Publishers. Academic Press, US (2002)
22. Marcus, A.: User-interface design, culture, and the future. In: AVI 2002: Proceedings of the Working Conference on Advanced Visual Interfaces. ACM (2002)
23. Mockups, `http://www.interaction-design.org/encyclopedia/mock-ups.html` (accessed February 24, 2011)

24. Rosson, M.B., Carroll, J.M.: Usability Engineering, Scenario-Based Development of Human-Computer Interaction. Morgan Kaufmann Publishers, Academic Press (2002)
25. Garrett, J.J.: The elements of user experience: user-centered design for the web. AIGA, Berkeley (2003)
26. Paratala, T., Kangaskirte, R.: The Combined Walkthrough: Measuring Behavioral, Affective, and Cognitive Information in Usability Testing. Journal of Usability Studies 5(1), 21–33 (2009)
27. Zheng, Z.: Overview of usability evaluation methods, http://www.usabilityhome.com (accessd August 16, 2010)
28. Ikonen, V., Kaasinen, E., Niemelä, M., Leikas, J.: Ethical Guidelines for Mobile-Centric Ambient Intelligence, Tech. Rep., (2008), http://www.fp6-minami.org/fileadmin/user/pdf/WS/MINAmI_D14_EthicalguidelinesforAmI.pdf
29. Pekkola, M., Jantunen, I., Wang, X., Korhonen, T., Vatanen, M.: An Online Social Networking Service as a Source of Support and Health Information – A Study on Users Experiences. In: eHealth 2010, Casablanca, Morocco, December 13-15 (2010)
30. Mallenius, S., Rossi, M., Tuunainen, V.K.: Factors affecting the adoption and use of mobile devices and services by elderly people – results from a pilot study
31. Life-Link Active Alert Call service & Medical Alert System, http://www.callforassistance.com/index.html (accessed August 16, 2010)
32. Remote Alert Emergency Call System from Independent Living Center, http://www.ilcnsw.asn.au/items/2861 (accessd August 16, 2010)
33. Medical Alert, http://www.medicalalert.com/ (accessed September 01, 2010)
34. Statistics Finland: Injuries Cause by Falls the Most Common Reason for Fatal Accidents (February 22, 2011), http://www.stat.fi/til/ksyyt/2009/01/ksyyt_2009_01_2011-02-22_tie_001_en.html
35. Atun, R.A., Sittampalam, S.R., Mohan, A.: Uses and Benefits of SMS in Health-care Delivery
36. Life Guardian, http://www.lifeguardianmedicalalarms.com/ accessed September 02, 2010)
37. Falls Among Older Adults: An Overview, http://www.cdc.gov/HomeandRecreationalSafety/Falls/adultfalls.html (accessed September 02, 2010)
38. Alertacall, http://www.alertacall.com/ (accessed August 17, 2010)

Estimating Older People's Physical Functioning with Automated Health Monitoring Technologies at Home: Feature Correlations and Multivariate Analysis

Juho Merilahti, Juha Pärkkä, and Ilkka Korhonen

VTT, Tekniikankatu 1, PO Box 1300, 33101, Tampere, Finland
{Juho.Merilahti,Juha.Parkka}@vtt.fi, Ilkka.Korhonen@tut.fi

Abstract. As person's functional capacity determines partly one's independency and quality of life, it should be observed and monitored. We calculated different features from actigraphy, bed sensor, pedometer, weight scale and blood pressure monitor over time period varying between one and two weeks. These features' connections to typical functional capacity tests such as ADL, balance and muscle strength were studied. No single feature was connected to all the functioning measures which again suggest importance of screening multiple health data sources. Created multivariate model to estimate holistic functional status has statistically significant correlation with ADL and two lower limb muscle strength tests, and almost statistically significant correlation with balance and walk tests.

Keywords: Physical functioning, actigraphy, bed sensor, pedometer, weight scale, blood pressure monitor.

1 Introduction

Current demographic change (i.e. portion of the older adults in community is growing) is causing a lack of resources and drives the research at new innovative solutions for securing successful aging. Although theoretical model of "successful aging" is not unambiguous, physical functioning is one main factor of it [1,2]. Verbrugge and Jette in 1994 (in Cress [3]) wrote that "Functional capacity can be defined as an individual's inherent capability to perform fundamental physical, emotional and mental actions." Hence, physical functioning status describes how able one is to perform daily routines physically i.e. live independently when physical aspects are considered. Masala and Petretto concluded that newest models of disability (causes lack in independency) take into account both the person and the environment [4]. However, currently the environment (including different assisting instruments) cannot compensate all the functional deficits and good physical functioning is a corner stone of the independent living.

According to Cress it is necessary for primary and secondary prevention of disabilities to screen, assess and objectively measure physical functioning. Cress reported that measures are needed to discriminate the functional status and change in that status in different stage of health and age. Fundamental qualities for these measures are

M. Rautiainen et al. (Eds.): GPC 2011 Workshops, LNCS 7096, pp. 94–104, 2012.

test-retest reproducibility, validity, and sensitivity to change in the functional status [3]. Fig. 1 presents roughly a model described by Hickey (in [3]) for functional decline and a diagnostic criterion according to some evaluation metric. Although there are well studied and validated instruments and measures for different levels of functional decline the identification of preclinical state of disability would be important (one example of such a state in Fig. 1).

Nowadays different low cost technologies such as accelerometers provide a mean to record objectively subject's health behavior in long term conditions. For example Karnik and Mazzatti concluded that these technologies should "be validated against a battery of currently used—and widely accepted—techniques and indices" [5]; in this context physical functioning tests. Carvalho-Bos et al [6] and Paavilainen et al [7] found interesting correlation between actigraphy based features and functional status of demented subjects which implies that long term monitoring technologies could give important information automatically from the person's functional status.

In this paper we study health monitoring technologies' performance to estimate physical functioning level evaluated with widely used clinical instruments. The focus is on the preclinical state. We hypothesize that health data of older people with varying physical functioning status would give indication how the measured variables would change in very long term setup when the functioning would change as well.

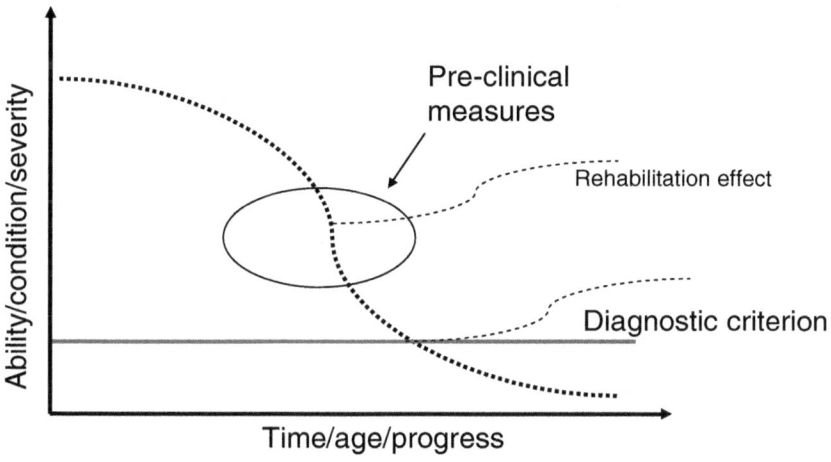

Fig. 1. Model for functional decline, clinical (diagnostic criterion) and pre-clinical measures

2   Methods

2.1   Subjects and Material

The study group consists of older people who live in an assisted living facility which provides accommodation and rehabilitation services for older and disabled people. During the study the subjects participated in a health intervention designed to increase their physical activity (Fig. 2). In the study health related data were collected with different technologies at the subjects' homes. The inclusion criteria for the subjects were: volunteering to participate in the intervention and the study, having self-reported sleep problems, loneliness or low physical activity level. The exclusion criteria were: having an acute disease, being in the active degeneration phase of a chronic disease, having a known disturbing event like a surgery during the study, a neurological disorder which prevented subject from using the system's components, dementia, any physical limitation that prevented their participation in the guided physical exercise, or depression without a medication. The study was approved by the appropriate ethics committee. The 19 older people (14 females, see Table 1) took part in the study. The average participation period was 84 days (range 19–107).

Functioning Measures

Before the three-month study period, a gerontologist interviewed the participants and collected material from subjects' functioning and health. The material is used as a reference. For the analysis we included:

- Mini mental state examination (**MMSE**); 0 to 30 (30 for no memory problems)
- Basic and instrumental activities of daily living (**ADL**): 15 to 60 (15 for totally independent)
- Geriatric depression scale (**GDS-15**); 0 (no depression) to 15 (15 for extreme depression)
- Sleeping pill usage; <yes, no>; mainly for controlling sleep and circadian (diurnal) rhythm related features in the analysis.

In the beginning and in the end of the study, a physiotherapist evaluated the participants' functioning via several tests. These measures are used as a reference as well. The test set is partly based on the set developed by State Treasury of Finland for evaluating veterans' functioning [8] and partly on Berg Balance Scale [9]. There exist reference values for finish older population for most of the tests [8]. The items included in the analysis are (see also Table 1):

- Hand grip test of both hands (**Hand grip**); results depends especially on gender according to [8]
- Time for five chair rises (**Chair rises**); age and gender do not have major effect on the result [8]
- Crouch times (**Crouches**): crouching as many times one can (max 50 times); depends on gender, but good reference values for older people are missing
- Walking speed of 10 meters (**Walk test**); age and gender do not have major effect on the result [8]
- **Balance** test; standing with feet together , retrieving object from floor, turning 360 degrees, tandem stance, standing on one foot – derived from Berg Balance Scale, (scale 0-20; worst-best). According to reference values in [9] age and gender do not have major effect on the result

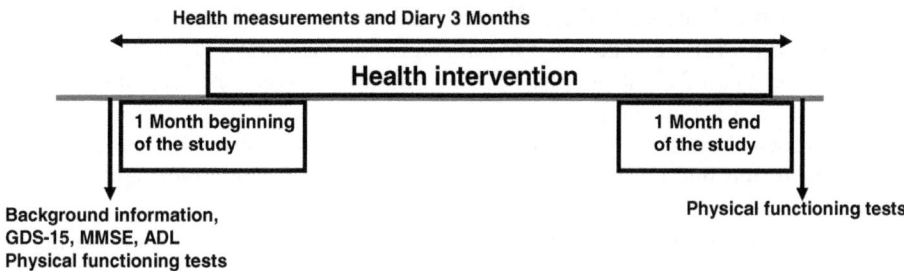

Fig. 2. The study description

Table 1. Demographics and physical functioning test results

Variable	N	Mean	Standard deviation	Range [min max]
Age	19	78	7.8	[60-86]
MMSE	16	27.5	3.3	[18 30]
ADL	19	20.3	6.7	[14 40]
GDS-15	19	1.9	1.6	[0 5]
Hand grip(right/left)	19/19	22.3/22.4	8.3/9.8	[10 46]/[9 47]
Chair rises [sec]	19	11.3	3.1	[6.5 17.6]
Crouches	19	27.9	16	[4 50]
Walk test [sec]	19	8.4	1.9	[5.3 12.9]
Balance	19	15.2	3.3	[8 20]

Health Technologies

The data from different health technologies were collected automatically and with a paper diary. The technologies were.

1) Actigraphy: Vivago is a wrist-worn wireless activity monitor (IST WristCare, Vivago, Helsinki, Finland, similar to actigraphy; www.istsec.fi) and can observe a person's activity and sleep/wake patterns 24/7. The method has been reported to perform sleep/wake classification with similar accuracy to actigraphy, which is the most commonly used alternative to polysomnography in sleep analysis. The Vivago is reported to be highly sensitive to detect self-reported naps as well [10].

2) Bed sensor: Vital signs during the bed time were collected using an electromechanical film sensor (Emfit Ltd, Vaajakoski, Finland; www.emfit.com). The bed sensor was installed below the user's mattress. The device detects time spend in bed with one minute resolution. It also infers heart rate, breathing frequency and strength of activity for each minute.

3) Steps: Omron Walking Style II pedometer was used to collect daily step count which the subjects wrote down in the paper diary.

4) Weight: OBH Nordica Weight scale results were collected to the diary (subjects were instructed to measure the weight in the morning)

5) Morning and evening blood pressure: Omron 705IT, the diary

We had two problems with the automated data collection during the study. 1) A wrong log off procedure shut down the manager software and caused six weeks loss of bed sensor data of eight people. 2) The actigraphy's software for collecting data was located on a server computer at the facility. For an unknown reason the server was shut down during the summer vacation (most likely caused by the renovation work done in the building), causing a four-week loss of actigraphy data for seven subjects.

In addition to above mentioned problems due the subjects' usage or measuring behavior the collected data had some missing values (compliance and data collection are described in more details in [11]). For feature calculation we manually selected one to two weeks period from the beginning of the study including as good data as possible i.e. minimizing missing values and excluding technical failure periods. Features including at least seven days of data (length was narrowed to maximum 14 days) are use in the analysis.

2.2   Data Processing

Features
From the good quality data (seven to 14 days) we calculated or selected the following features for the analysis. The selection of the features is based on our earlier experience [7, 12 and 13]. For continuous features (actigraphy and bed sensor) the daily data (21:00-21:00) were divided to day (10:00-20:00) and to night (00:00-06:00). A mean is calculated from the daily features for each subject.

1) Actigraphy features for each day (median is used as the data are not normally distributed):

- Median of activity data during the circadian period (**Circ median**): daily data including more than 10 hours of data are included, see out of range feature
- Median of activity data during the day (**Day median**): days including more than 3 hours of data are included
- Median of activity data during the night (**Night median**):nights including more than 3 hours of data are included
- Daytime sleep/passive time (**Day sleep**): The actigraphy's software's minute-to-minute sleep/wake classification information is aggregated over day time. The sleep class represents sleep or passivity.
- Sleep time (**Night sleep**): The software provides the time slept at night
- Circadian rhythm strength from the software (**Circ rhythm**): The feature is calculated by dividing night time average activity (within 11pm – 5am) with day time average activity (between 8am – 8pm). The values varies between zero and ten, ten represent good circadian rhythm.
- Out of base station range (**Out of range**): The system detects when the wrist unit is outside the range of the base station. However, the activity data is not available during these periods. Out of range feature is sum of minutes person has spend outside the range during the day. This means that for active

persons (i.e. spending lot of time outside home) significant amount of activity data can be missing which might distort the day time actigraphy features.

2) Bed sensor (nights when bed was occupied at least three hours are included). Features are calculated for the periods the bed was occupied:

- Standard deviation of night time signal amplitude (**Night amplSD**): tells about the restlessness (amplitude is proportional to pressure against the sensor i.e. related subject's body mass)
- Mean night time heart rate (**Night HR**)
- Mean night time breathing frequency (**Night breathfreq**)

3) **Steps**

4) **Weight**

5) Systolic and diastolic blood pressure at evening and morning (**Bpsys mor, Bpdia mor, Bpsys eve** and **Bpdia eve**)

Statistical Analysis

Visual observations via Scatter plot and statistical via Spearman rank correlation (as the number of the subjects was small) are used to discover connection between calculated features and functioning measures. We also calculated partial correlates (Spearman) controlled for age, gender and sleeping pill usage.

We coded the hand grip test's results to worse (-1), equal (0) or better (1) as the reference values are heavily related to age and gender. If the result of a subject differed over 2 kg from the reference it was given either -1 or 1. ADL, balance, hand grip factors, crouches and chair rise were used to create clusters with K-Means clustering method. We assume that these clusters would represent subjects with different functioning status. The selection of suitable number of clusters is done by observing number of cases in each cluster for reasonable distribution and centroids. We assume that combination of different tests gives a holistic picture of person's functioning status. GDS-15 was excluded as it represents more the mental functioning than physical. The feature correlations are studied against these cluster results as well. Linear regression with backward selection method is utilized with the most promising features for studying multivariate model's performance to estimate the persons functioning. Adjusted R square is utilized to describe the model's goodness of fit. SPSS (17.0) and Matlab (R2009a) environments are used in the data analysis.

3   Results

MMSE results are removed from the analysis because of a small variance (ceiling effect of the instrument) in the study group (only one demented person participated in the study; her husband aided with the technology). Table 2 presents Spearman correlation between the features and the physical functioning test results. Also connections with $P < 0.1$ are presented as the number of cases is small. Table 2 contains also the partial correlations controlled for age, gender and sleeping pill usage.

Table 2. Spearman correlation (rho) between the features and functioning tests. Values in the parenthesis are partial correlations controlled for age, gender and sleeping pill usage.

	GDS-15	ADL	Balance	Crouches	Chair rise time	Walk speed
Circ median				0.52 (0.57) N=14	-0.58* (-0.66*) N=14	
Day median				0.53 (0.58) N=15	-0.58* (-0.67*) N=15	
Night median				0.53* N=14	-0.48 (0.53) N=14	
Day sleep				-0.72** (-0.69*) N=15	0.50 N=14	
Night sleep				-0.56* (-0.56) N=13	0.50 (0.53) N=14	
Circ rhythm						
Out of range		-0.67** N=14		0.49 (0.61) N=13		
Night amplSD		-0.48 (-0.69) N=14	0.56* N=14			-0.63* N=14
Night HR		-0.69** (-0.80**) N=14			(-0.58) N=14	-0.52 (-0.69*) N=14
Nigth breatfreq						
Steps	-0.66** (-0.51) N=18	-0.56* (-0.52*) N=18	0.55* N=18		-0.42 N=18	-0.58* (0.56*) N=18
Weight	0.42 N=19					(0.48) N=18
Bpsys/Bpdia mor						
Bpsys/Bpdia eve	0.40/- N=18	(0.52*/-) N=18				

*P < 0.05 (without marker P < 0.1).
**P < 0.01.

In case of two clusters in K-Means clustering the study group is divided evenly (N=9 for both clusters); one functioning test value was missing. Only **Out of range** feature differs statistically significantly (P < 0.05), and **Day sleep** has almost statistically significant difference (P < 0.1) between the two clusters according to Mann-Whitney U-test. Table 3 presents the clusters' centroids.

For four clusters case there are 5-7-4-2 cases in each cluster after the clusters are ordered according to functioning status (the first cluster with five cases having the best functioning status). The ordered cluster number is selected to represent the holistic physical functioning status (1=best, 4=worse). According to Spearman correlation analysis **Day sleep** (RHO=0.57, P<0.05) **Day median** (RHO=-0.55, P<0.05) and **Out of range** (RHO=-0.66, P<0.05) have statistically significant correlation with the four clusters. **Circ median** and **Steps** had almost statistically significant correlation (P < 0.1).

Table 3. Two and four clusters' centroids for functioning tests according to K-Means clustering

Variable	Two clusters		Four clusters			
Cluster ordinal	1	2	1	2	3	4
Walk test	9.2	7.7	7.8	8.1	9.3	9.6
Chair rises	12.8	9.7	9.1	9.9	16.0	12.3
Crouches	15	41	50	26	9	17
Balance	14	17	18	15	13	14
ADL	23	18	16	19	19	35
Hand grip right	-0.56	-0.56	-0.40	-0.86	-0.25	-0.50
Hand grip left	-0.44	-0.33	-0.20	-0.71	0.00	-0.50

Table 4. Features in multivariate models after linear regression with backward selection algorithm

Variable	GDS-15	ADL	Balance	Crouches	Chair rise	Walk speed	Cluster of four
Circ median				x			x
Day median		x					
Night median							
Day sleep					x	x	
Night sleep		x				x	
Out of range		x		x			x
Night amplSD			x	x		x	x
Night HR		x			x		
Steps	x	x		x			
Age		x	x	x			
Gender			x	x	x		
R square adjusted	0.34	0.82	0.73	0.65	0.55	0.47	0.65

All the features which have at least one statistically significant correlation and one almost statistically significant correlation with some of the physical functioning test results are included in the linear regression analysis together with gender and age. Missing values are replaced by group mean to maximize the number of cases in the analysis Table 4 presents which features remain in the model when the backward selection algorithm is utilized. We use $P<0.05$ as include criterion and $P>0.1$ as exclusion criterion for the backward selection method. Bias term was included. Fig. 3 visualizes an example of the model's output against four cluster result (rightmost column in Table 4).

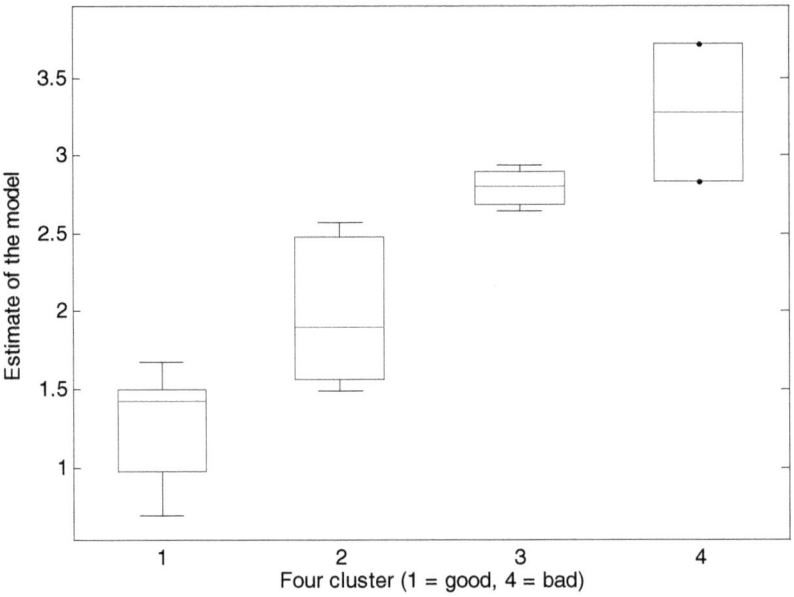

Fig. 3. Boxplot of multivariate linear model's output (rightmost column in Table 4) and four clusters of physical functioning

4   Discussion and Conclusions

We studied how health data measured via different health technologies are connected to functional status of an older person. The subjects' functional status contained variance according to used tests and we assume that the population represents well people who stand in the preclinical state (as in Fig. 1) when the diagnosis, a risk of losing independency according to the physical functioning. Two functional measures (MMSE and step height) were left out due to the ceiling effect. As a result we expected to propose an instrument which tells about the user's functional status and possible change in it, and can be monitored automatically during the normal daily life.

We found out that many selected features were connected with the reference functional measures and when controlling for age, gender and sleeping pill usage no major changes were observed in these connections. Somewhat surprising was that circadian rhythm strength did not have statistically significant correlation with the reference values as suchlike features are found to be heavily connected to functional status, although mainly with demented subjects [6,7]. One explanation for this distinction could be the reason that in [7] subjects involved were less independent i.e. worse functioning state. Another reason can be that in the current study some of the subjects (mainly ones with the good functioning) spend lot of time outside thus preventing the actigraphy to record activity during these periods. This has effect on the circadian rhythm value. This emphasizes the need to have a short term data logger at the wrist unit as activity data during these periods might be very relevant.

There were some unexpected connections of Night amplSD and Night median features with functional test results. The Night amplSD was found to correlate in same direction as steps although we expected that more restful the night would mean better functional status. More work is needed to find out right features for restlessness during the night.

No single feature was found to be connected to every functioning measure or included in the regression model, although steps was found to be very promising. This implies that it would be important to screen multiple sources to detect possible changes in the physical functioning. For example when analyzing the connection between functioning tests results and estimate developed against the four cluster reference, ADL, Crouches and Chair rise results were found to have statistically significant correlation, and Balance and Walk test almost significant correlation with the model which included three very distinctive features..

The findings are preliminary and more long-term data should be collected for studying this approach thoroughly. In addition we need to look into the properties such as test-retest reproducibility and sensitivity to change. The day time activity behavior measured via actigraphy should be collected over whole day as it was now partly missing due to the system properties. However, Out of range feature was found to be very interesting and might be a good addition to traditional Actigraphic features.

References

1. Bowling, A., Iliffe, S.: Which model of successful ageing should be used? Baseline findings from a British longitudinal survey of ageing. Age and Ageing 35(6), 607–614 (2006)
2. Cruz-Jentoft, A.J., Franco, A., Sommer, P., Baeyens, J.P., Jankowska, E., Maggi, A., Ponikowski, P., Ryś, A., Szczerbinska, K., Michel, J.-P., Milewicz, A.: Silver paper: The future of health promotion and preventive actions, basic research, and clinical aspects of age-related disease: A report of the European summit on age-related disease. Aging - Clinical and Experimental Research 21(6), 376–385 (2009)
3. Cress, M.E.: Assessment of physical performance in older adults. In: Poon, L.W., Chodzko –Zajko, W., Tomporowski, P.D. (eds.) Active Living, Cognitive Functioning, and Aging, HumanKinetics (2006)

4. Masala, C., Petretto, D.R.: From disablement to enablement: Conceptual models of disability in the 20th century. Disability and Rehabilitation 30(17), 1233–1244 (2008)
5. Karnik, K., Mazzatti, D.J.: Review of tools and technologies to assess multi-system functional impairment and frailty. Clinical Medicine: Geriatrics (3), 1–8 (2009)
6. Carvalho-Bos, S.S., Riemersma-van Der Lek, R.F., Waterhouse, J., Reilly, T., Van Someren, E.J.W.: Strong association of the rest-activity rhythm with well-being in demented elderly women. American Journal of Geriatric Psychiatry 15(2), 92–100 (2007)
7. Paavilainen, P., Korhonen, I., Lötjönen, J., Cluitmans, L., Jylhä, M., Särelä, A., et al.: Circadian activity rhythm in demented and non-demented nursing-home residents measured by telemetric actigraphy. Journal of Sleep Research 14(1), 61–68 (2005)
8. Hamilas M, Hämäläinen H, Koivunen M, Lähteenmäki L, Pajala S, Pohjola L.: Toimiva – testit. Iäkkäiden fyysisen toimintakyvyn mittausmenetelmä. Valtiokonttori, report of State Treasure's test set results (2000),
   http://www.valtiokonttori.fi/sove/Tarjousp_Toimiva.rtf
9. Steffen, T.M., Hacker, T.A., Mollinger, L.: Age- and gender-related test performance in communitydwelling elderly people: six-minute walk test, Berg balance scale, timed up & go test and gaitspeeds. Phys Ther. 82, 128–137 (2002)
10. Lötjönen, J., Korhonen, I., Hirvonen, K., Eskelinen, S., Myllymäki, M., Partinen, M.: Automatic sleep-wake and nap analysis with a new wrist worn online activity monitoring device Vivago WristCare. Sleep 26(1), 86–90 (2003)
11. Merilahti, J., Pärkkä, J., Antila, K., Paavilainen, P., Mattila, E., Malm, E.-J., Saarinen, A., Korhonen, I.: Compliance and technical feasibility of long-term health monitoring with wearable and ambient technologies. Journal of Telemedicine and Telecare 15(6), 302–309 (2009)
12. Pärkkä, J., Merilahti, J., Mattila, E.M., Malm, E., Antila, K., Tuomisto, M.T., Viljam Saarinen, A., van Gils, M., Korhonen, I.: Relationship of psychological and physiological variables in long-term self-monitored data during work ability rehabilitation program. IEEE Transactions on Information Technology in Biomedicine 13(2), 141–151 (2009)
13. Merilahti, J., Pärkkä, J., Korhonen, I.: Connections of daytime napping and vigilance measures to activity behaviour and physical functioning. Proceeding (723) Biomedical Engineering (2011)

Applying MTC and Femtocell Technologies to the Continua Health Reference Architecture

Edward Mutafungwa

Department of Communications and Networking, Aalto University
P.O. Box 13000, 00076 Aalto, Espoo, Finland
edward.mutafungwa@tkk.fi

Abstract. The Continua reference architecture is increasingly becoming the *de facto* framework for implementation of personal telehealth system. So far, the Continua guidelines have specified the use of personal or local area network technologies (Bluetooth, USB, ZigBee) for personal health device connectivity within the monitored person's local environment. However, there is growing interest in machine-type communications (MTC) and femtocell home gateways within the mobile communications domain, which could impact the implementation of systems for home services, such as, personal telehealth. Against this backdrop, this paper analyzes the potential added value, as well as challenges, in augmenting personal telehealth systems with Continua-compliant MTC personal health devices with integrated 3GPP interfaces (GPRS, HSPA, LTE etc.) and operating in a femtocell home network environment.

Keywords: Continua, Femtocells, Machine-Type Communications, Personal Telehealth, Home Networks.

1 Introduction

Personal telehealth services that enable proactive out-of-hospital patient-managed care can not only reduce the fast rising cost of healthcare, but also improve the quality of care [1]. The Continua Health Alliance[1] (henceforth, referred to simply as "Continua") is arguably the most prominent open industry group providing interoperability guidelines and certification programs for the implementation of personal telehealth systems. The Continua interoperability guidelines are developed from use cases (defining actors, actions, assumptions, etc.) that are derived across three intersecting personal telehealth application domains [2], namely: ageing independently; chronic disease management; and health and wellness.

The generated use cases form the basis for requirements specifications for Continua personal telehealth systems and assist in the identification of standards development organizations (SDOs) that produce standards that meet the system requirements. One notable SDO is the Third Generation Partnership Project (3GPP) that specifies standards for mobile communications (e.g. GSM, WCDMA/HSPA,

---

[1] Continua Health Alliance: http://www.continuaalliance.org/

M. Rautiainen et al. (Eds.): GPC 2011 Workshops, LNCS 7096, pp. 105–114, 2012.
© Springer-Verlag Berlin Heidelberg 2012

LTE etc.). The 3GPP has now extended the capability of mobile networks to efficiently cater for local radio access environments using femtocell technologies and connectivity to a wider range of end-user devices by virtue of Machine-Type Communications (MTC) paradigm. In this paper, we apply femtocell and MTC concepts to personal telehealth systems and identify how they could add value to future system implementations within the Continua framework. The remainder of the paper is organized as follows. Section 2 provides a brief description of the Continua reference architecture, while Section 3 introduces the MTC and femtocell concepts. Section 4 describes how the MTC and femtocell technologies could enhance Continua personal telehealth systems and also outlines existing challenges. Concluding remarks are then presented in Section 5.

2   Continua Reference Architecture

The Continua interoperability guidelines utilize the end-to-end Continua reference architecture to represent the high-level structure of the personal telehealth system and provide commonly-agreed terminology for different device classes and interfaces used within the system (see Figure 1) [2].

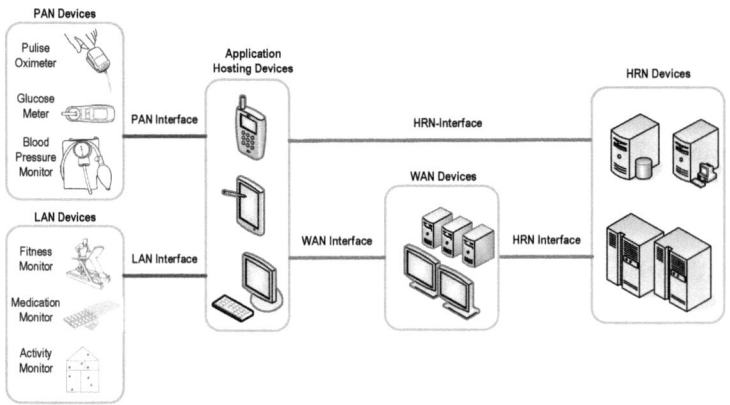

Notes: HRN = Health Reporting Network, LAN = Local Area Network, PAN = Personal Area Network, WAN = Wide Area Network

Fig. 1. Continua reference architecture

2.1   Continua Device Classes

Continua has defined the following health devices classes for the reference architecture: Personal Area Network (PAN) Device, Local Area Network (LAN) Devices, Application Hosting Device (AHD), Wide Area Network (WAN) Device and Health Reporting Network (HRN) Device classes (see Figure 1). The PAN devices typically refer to portable health sensors or actuators, such as, pulse oximeters, blood pressure monitors and glucose meters, which are worn, implanted or attached to the monitored person, or alternatively deployed within close proximity (few meters) of the person. On the other hand, LAN devices are sensors or actuators that may have a relatively larger form factor (e.g., fitness equipment) or are embedded in the monitored person's home environment (e.g., independent living activity sensors). The AHD is a user device (e.g., mobile handset, tablet PC, set-top-box) that aggregates data from PAN and LAN devices, provides a gateway to WAN or HRN devices, and may itself also implement some health sensing or actuation functionality.

The WAN and HRN devices are typically deployed by telehealth service providers or care givers in geographically separate locations from the monitored person's home environment. A WAN device could be an application or web server platform that collects data from personal health devices (PAN, LAN or AHD devices) and provisions a telehealth service (e.g., remote fitness trainer). The HRN devices are typically information repositories, such as, a hospital's Electronic Medical Records (EMR) or patient's Personal Health Records (PHR), which sit on the boundary of the personal telehealth system and facilitate the exchange of patient-centric information with the WAN or AHD devices.

2.2   Continua Interfaces

The Continua reference architecture currently defines four main interfaces (PAN, LAN, WAN and HRN interfaces) between different device classes as depicted in Figure 1. The Continua PAN interface currently utilizes Bluetooth and Universal Serial Bus (USB) for wireless and wireline data transport, respectively, while ZigBee is has been defined for wireless data transport in the LAN interface. Both the PAN and LAN interfaces use a transport-independent data exchange protocol adapted from the Institute of Electrical and Electronics Engineers (IEEE) 11073 Personal Health Data (PHD)[2] standards family (see Figure 2). These include the baseline IEEE 11073-20601 standard which defines application layer services (e.g., connection

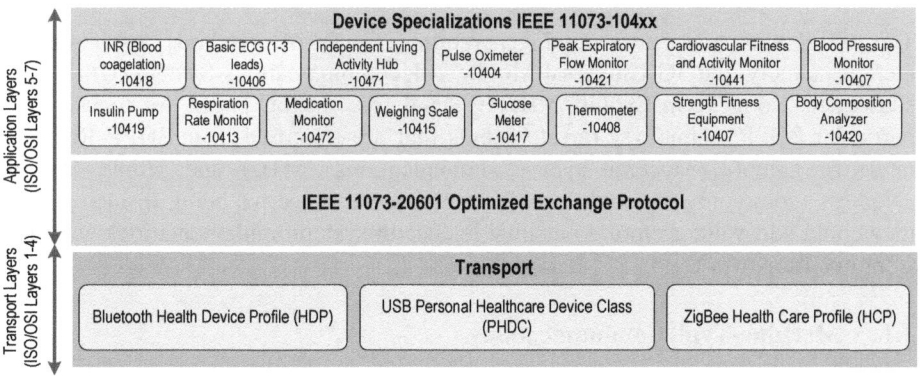

Fig. 2. IEEE 11073 personal health device conceptual framework. Note: device specializations in yellow boxes are still under development.

---

[2] IEEE 11073 PHD WG: http://standards.ieee.org/develop/wg/WG-11073-104xx.html

management, reliable data transfer) and an optimized data exchange protocol (e.g., commands, device configuration information, interoperable data format etc.) over the PAN and LAN interfaces [3]. Each PAN or LAN personal health device (see Figure 2) has a corresponding IEEE 11073-104xx specification (where xx is any number from 01 to 99) to describe how it utilizes IEEE 11073-20601 to fulfill its functions. Different industry alliances and SDOs have partnered with the Continua alliance to produce customized versions of their standard protocol stacks by including support for IEEE 11073 for use in personal telehealth systems (e.g. Bluetooth HDP [4]).

The WAN and HRN interfaces describes the connection between personal health devices (PAN, LAN and AHD devices) and devices in the clinical domain (WAN and HRN devices). For both interfaces, the Continua alliance opted for alignment with the Integrating the Healthcare Enterprise (IHE) initiative[3] that is the leading promoter of standards from bodies, such as, Healthcare Layer 7 (HL7), for use in the clinical domain. For the WAN interface, Continua uses the PCD-01 transactions of the IHE Device Enterprise Communication (DEC) profile to transform IEEE 11073 personal health device data into the widely used HL7 2.x message format (while retaining IEEE 11073 semantics) and then uses Web Services (IHE IT Infrastructure standard) for sending the data to target WAN device(s) [2]. The HRN interface uses IEEE 11073 or other semantics (e.g., SNOMED-CT[4]) and the XML-based HL7 Clinical Document Architecture (CDA) with a customized Performance Healthcare Monitoring Report (PHMR) document format to accommodate personal health device monitoring [2]. The actual data transport in the HRN interface may be based on Web Services (IHE Cross-Enterprise Document Reliable Interchange, XDR) or simply email (IHE Cross-Enterprise Document Media Interchange, XDM) [2].

3   3GPP Architectural Enhancements

The 3GPP maintains the second generation (2G) GSM standards and evolutions thereof, namely, the 3G Universal Mobile Telecommunications System (UMTS) and subsequent Long Term Evolution (LTE) standards. In this paper, we focus on two particular 3GPP technology developments that are specified from 3GPP Release 8 onwards, namely, Machine-Type Communications (MTC) and Home NodeBs/eNodeBs (commonly referred to as femtocells), the objective being to identify how they could add value to future personal telehealth system implementations within the Continua framework.

3.1   Machine-Type Communications

The smart home vision is one of information gathering and processing functionality embedded in everyday objects and interacting pervasively with the home dwellers [5]. Mobile network operators and equipment manufacturers are looking to contribute to

---

[3] Integrating the Healthcare Enterprise: http://www.ihe.net/
[4] Systematized Nomenclature of Medicine-Clinical Terms:
http://www.ihtsdo.org/snomed-ct/

this vision by extending network services from human-to-human (H2H) communications (via mobile phones, tablets etc.) to more general machine-type communications (MTC), whereby, MTC devices (e.g. smart meters, fitness monitors, etc.) may send/receive data autonomously to/from other MTC devices (or systems) via public mobile networks [6].

The MTC communication standards are currently being developed by, among others, the 3GPP [7], [9], [10] and the European Telecommunications Standards Institute (ETSI)[5] where the alternative term machine-to-machine communications (M2M) is used. The MTC standardization activities in 3GPP are closely aligned to those of ETSI M2M, but with the 3GPP standards having a narrower scope by focusing mostly on 3GPP radio access and core networks, between MTC devices and the edge nodes of the 3GPP core network. The health use cases have been described in both 3GPP MTC [7] and ETSI M2M working groups [8], and are considered to be one of the main future drivers for MTC/M2M. The discussion in the rest of the paper focuses on 3GPP standardized MTC technologies, but the observations made could be equally applicable to other non-3GPP M2M technologies (WiMAX, WiFi, satellite, CDMA2000, DSL, etc.) being considered within the ETSI framework.

3.2   Residential Femtocell Networks

Femtocells have recently emerged as an attractive solution for boosting network coverage and achieving quality-of-service (QoS) for subscribers in indoor environments [12], without the need for costly upgrades to the conventional macrocellular network [11]. Femtocellular networks consist of inexpensive plug-and-play femto base stations or femtocells that can be deployed autonomously by subscriber in a residential or enterprise premises, in a similar manner to Digital Subscriber Line (DSL) or cable modems. Each deployed femto base station is then backhauled via the wireline broadband access link (e.g. xDSL twisted-pair line) available locally in the site of deployment to a femto gateway node and the mobile operator core network. Access to femtocellular services (voice, mobile data etc.) is usually restricted to a closed subscriber group (CSG), such as, household members.

The development of femtocell technologies is currently ongoing within 3GPP and industry consortia (e.g. Femto Forum), as well as, other key SDOs maintaining parallel mobile network standards (3GPP2, IEEE 802.16 etc.). In the 3GPP standards, femto base stations that operate in the UMTS and LTE environments are known as, Home Node Bs (HNBs) and Home eNodeBs (HeNBs), respectively [12]. These labels provide a distinction from the respective 3GPP NodeB and eNodeB terms used for UMTS and LTE macro base stations.

4   Adapting MTC and Femtocells for the Continua Framework

4.1   MTC Devices as Personal Health Devices

Legacy Continua personal health devices utilize PAN/LAN technologies (Bluetooth, ZigBee and USB) for data transport. Recently, an agreement was reached between the

---

[5] ETSI M2M communications: `http://www.etsi.org/Website/Technologies/M2M.aspx`

Continua and the Global Certification Forum (GCF)[6] to promote development and oversee certification of Continua health devices embedded with 3GPP (GSM, WCDMA, HSPA, LTE etc.) wireless modules.   The latter GCF agreement is particularly significant as it extends direct connectivity of Continua certified devices beyond the PAN/LAN domain by virtue of 3GPP wireless connectivity and exposes the mobile operators' services and selected assets for development of numerous new applications for Continua use cases. Specifically the following benefits are envisioned:

Subscriber Data Management: Mobile network operators maintain several repositories for subscriber-related data, such as, the Authorization, Authentication and Accounting (AAA) servers; Equipment Identity Register (EIR) servers; and the Home Subscriber Servers (HSS) which holds the subscriber profiles, service permissions, preferences, location information and usage histories. To that end, mobile operators provide application programming interfaces (APIs) that enable third party providers (e.g., personal telehealth service providers) to build innovative applications based on this valuable data [13].   From the Continua personal telehealth system perspective, this should facilitate addition of Continua certified MTC personal health devices to the mobile subscribers profile, creation of device-specific access policies, utilization of carrier-grade security features, and enable useful interaction between personal telehealth services and other personal services (home security, social media, etc.).

Remote Device Management: Mobile device management standards, such as, Open Mobile Alliance (OMA) Device Management (DM)[7] allow personal telehealth service providers (or system operators) to have remote management access to personal health devices in patient's environment, enabling functionality, such as, remote parameter configuration, device fault management, service (de)activation and software/firmware upgrades.

Quality of Service, Charging and Policy Control: The evolving mobile core network is offering increasingly sophisticated ways for differentiation of both services and subscribers [14]. Data bearers provide end-to-end logical transport for IP traffic across mobile networks and each bearer is assigned QoS parameters (e.g., guaranteed bit rates, packet delay, packet error rate, priority etc.) that enable differentiation in treatment of traffic flows from different services (e.g., health data flows versus non-health data) during admission control and resource allocation. The introduction of Policy Control and Charging (PCC) functionality in 3GPP Release 8 systems provides even more advanced QoS differentiation operating at the relatively fine-grained per-service session level rather than on a per-bearer level [14].   This could, for instance, enable differentiation amongst telehealth services according to their criticality

---

[6] The GCF operates an independent certification programme to help ensure global interoperability between 3GPP standardized mobile devices and networks. See GFC press release of 9 February 2011 on partnership with Continua:
http://www.globalcertificationforum.org/WebSite/public/continua.aspx

[7] OMA DM Working Group:
http://www.openmobilealliance.org/Technical/DM.aspx

(e.g., prioritizing ambulatory data over other non-critical health data). The PCC also includes functionality for both real-time online charging and offline charging, which could result in many alternative billing mechanisms and new innovative personal telehealth business models. For instance, from generated Charging Data Records (CDR) it is possible to identify which part of the personal telehealth service should be billed to the patient, and which is billed to their health insurance provider or local authority.

In order for personal telehealth systems to reap these aforementioned MTC benefits, a number of key technical challenges related to general implementation of MTC systems has to be addressed [9][10]. The notable challenges include:

***Signaling Congestion and Overload*:** The anticipated wave of MTC device proliferation [6] may disrupt the control plane by overloading core network nodes (SGSN/MME, GGSN/PGW, etc.) and congest signaling links due to MTC-related signaling (for mobility, recurring or simultaneous connection/attach requests etc.). A number of solutions are currently under study [10], such as, selective detachment of MTC devices or deactivation of bearers, scheduling of certain MTC traffic to off-peak times and exploitation of stationary or low mobility nature of most MTC device groups (e.g., most MTC personal health devices rarely used outside home) to minimize signaling related to mobility management procedures and paging.

***Addressing and Identifiers*:** The large number of MTC devices also presents a significant challenge in devising unique addresses for each individual device. With significant majority of MTC devices expected to subscribe to 3GPP packet-switched data services, the combination of the 15-digit International Mobile Subscriber Identifiers (IMSI) and IP addresses (mostly using IPv6 addressing rather than the limited IPv4 address space) appears to be the solution favored by most ongoing studies [10].

***Power Consumption*:** Devices using technologies, such as, ZigBee and Low Energy Bluetooth, have managed to achieve significant efficiencies in terms of power consumption by the going into sleep mode during periods of inactivity [16]. Furthermore, the range of indoor PAN/LAN radio links tend be few meters or 10s meters between paired devices or gateway, which means low device transmit powers are needed to compensate for distant-dependent path loss, resulting in more power saving. By contrast, MTC devices using 3GPP technologies would have shorter sleep cycles due to more frequent signaling operations, although this latter challenge is also addressed by the signaling optimization solutions mentioned previously. Furthermore, the 3GPP radio access links from indoor MTC devices usually terminate at an outdoor macro base station typically located kilometers away. This means in order to achieve radio performance targets (e.g., Signal to Interference and Noise Ratio) higher MTC device transmit powers are needed to overcome the higher distant-dependent path losses, shadowing (due to buildings, hills etc.) and co-channel interference.

4.2   Femtocells as a Home Gateway for Personal Telehealth Systems

Household member(s) dwelling in a smart would typically subscriber to multiple MTC services (telehealth, smart metering, home entertainment etc.), which may necessitate the management of multiple home networks, with each having its own gateway. The introduction of converged home M2M gateways is viewed as way of horizontal integration of disparate networks and simplifying network management [16]. Femtocell technologies provide an attractive way for implementing the converged gateway for the 3GPP MTC-based personal telehealth system described in previous Section. Figure 3 illustrates a simplified end-to-end high-level view of heterogeneous macrocell and femtocell deployments (radio access and core networks) to support a Continua personal telehealth system.

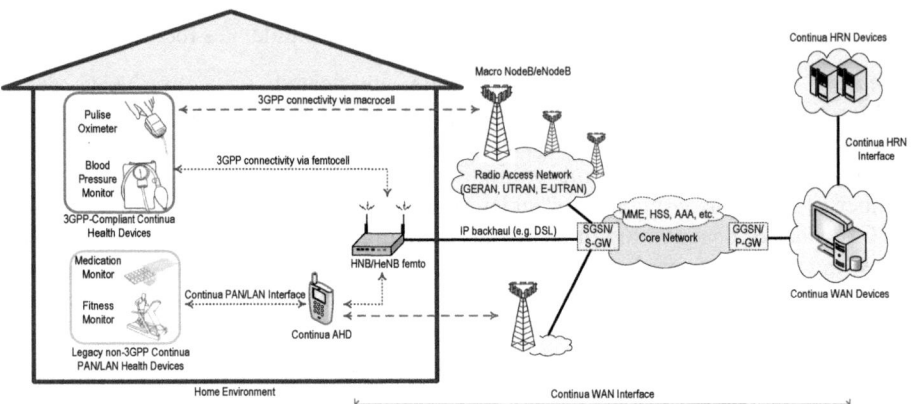

Notes: AAA = Accounting, Authentication and Authorization, AHD = Application Hosting Device, DSL = Digital Subscriber Line, E-UTRAN = Evolved UMTS RAN, GERAN = GSM Edge Radio Access Network, GGSN = Gateway GPRS Support Node, GPRS = General Packet Radio Service, GSM = Global System for Mobile, HRN = Health Reporting Network, HSS = Home Subscriber Server, IP = Internet Protocol, LAN = Local Area Network, LTE = Long Term Evolution, MME = Mobility Management Entity, PAN = Personal Area Network, P-GW = Packet Data Network Gateway, RAN = Radio Access Network, SGSN = Serving GPRS Support Node, S-GW = Serving Gateway, UMTS = Universal Mobile Telecommunications System, UTRAN = UMTS RAN, WAN = Wide Area Network, WCDMA = Wideband Code Division Multiple Access, 3GPP = Third Generation Partnership Project.

Fig. 3. High-level view of MTC and femtocell utilization for implementing the Continua personal telehealth system

The deployment of femtocell as home gateways presents a number benefits that positively impact the implementation of MTC services for systems, such as, the Continua personal telehealth system. These benefits include:

***Carrier-Grade Network Management and Security*:** Although femtocells are consumer devices autonomously deployed by a subscriber, they are actually managed by the operator. This enables advanced resource management and enhanced security by extending CSG restrictions to MTC devices. Furthermore, bringing network management functions closer to the managed MTC device entities alleviates the signaling load towards the mobile core network.

***Reduced Power Consumption*:** Femtocells are usually deployed locally in home environment (< 100m from MTC devices), leading to relatively low losses (propagation losses, wall attenuations etc.) and, hence, less device uplink transmit power requirements. This enables longer battery life or reduced grid power consumption compared to macrocellular case.

***Improved Indoor Coverage and Capacity*:** Femtocells enable superior indoor coverage compared to conventional macrocellular coverage, especially on the edge of the macrocell coverage areas [12]. This ensures service availability in all areas of the house (even in basements, attic, etc. which are usually macro coverage dead spots). Furthermore, femtocells offer relatively larger capacities (in both uplink and downlink) and avoid capacity drops due to fluctuating load conditions. This is attributed to the fact that, unlike macrocells, the femtocell usage is typically restricted to a private CSG. This scalable capacity could potentially enable wide area connectivity of personal health devices producing rich multimedia observations (e.g. high-resolution image fall sensors).

Multiple Radio Interfaces: Typical multi-radio femtocell designs include both 3GPP and non-3GPP interfaces, thus enabling compatibility with a diverse range of devices (sensors, actuators, mobile handsets etc.). An example is the Argela femtocell product[8] that integrates both 3GPP (WCDMA/HSPA) and non-3GPP (WiFi, ZigBee) interfaces. Furthermore, the availability of standard 3GPP interfaces by default on femtocells means that during femto downtime (e.g., due to power outage, backhaul link failure etc.) the 3GPP-compliant MTC devices may be handed over to the macrocell as a fallback measure ensuring service continuity for more critical telehealth applications.

Femtozone Applications: The Femto Forum Services Special Interest Group (SIG) has specified an API that exposes femtocell awareness information (presence, location or context) of devices and/or subscribers within the femto coverage areas [17]. Personal telehealth service developers may utilize the femto awareness API to provide innovate "femtozone applications" that add-value to the Continua use cases. For instance, a virtual fridge note application may prompt the femtocell to send medicine reminders only when the patient's returns to home environment (detected by inbound handover of patient's handset). Another example is a workflow enhancement application, whereby, detection of a visiting caregiver's handset entering the patient's femto coverage area would enable the patient's health context data to be automatically updated/activated on the caregiver's handset.

5   Conclusions and Future Work

This paper analyzed the potential beneficial impacts and challenges of 3GPP MTC and femtocells to the implementation of Continua personal telehealth system. It is clear that the aforementioned 3GPP mobile network enhancements could provide enhancements to Continua personal telehealth use cases. A closer analysis of the ongoing developments in MTC and femtocell standardization would enable personal telehealth system developers to produce systems that fully leverage the new features (e.g. Local IP Access breakout [18]) defined in those standards.

From the 3GPP wireless network engineering perspective, the performance in the local femtocellular environment is mainly limited by interference from neighboring femtocells, user equipment, macrocells and the increasing number of MTC devices. Therefore, research should address how interference mitigation techniques (power control optimization, beam forming, etc.) and Radio Resource Management (RRM)

---

[8] Argela Femtocell and Home Gateway:
http://www.argela.com/solutions.php?cid=femtocell

algorithms (for admission or flow control, dynamic scheduling, link adaptation etc.), could boost air interface resource utilization, reduce device power consumption and simultaneously meet the diverse QoS targets of personal telehealth services in the home environment.

Acknowledgments. This work was prepared in MOTIVE UBI-SERV project supported by the Academy of Finland (grant number 129446); and the CELTIC HOMESNET (CP6-009) project supported in part by the TEKES, NSN and ECE.

References

1. Gartner: eHealth for a Healthier Europe! – Opportunities for a Better Use of Healthcare Resources. Study on behalf of The Ministry of Health and Social Affairs in Sweden (2009)
2. Wartena, F., Muskens, J., Schmitt, L., Petković, M.: Continua: The Reference Architecture of a Personal Telehealth Ecosystem. In: Proceedings of the 12th IEEE International Conference on e-Health Networking Applications and Services (Healthcom), Lyon, p. 6 (2010)
3. ISO/IEEE 11073-20601: Health Informatics — Personal Health Device Communication —Part 20601: Application Profile — Optimized Exchange Protocol (2010)
4. Bluetooth SIG: Health Device Profile Specification. Version 1.0 (2008)
5. Chan, M., Campo, E., Esteve, D., Fournois, J.–Y.: Smart Homes – Current Features and Future Perspectives. Maturitas 64, 90–97 (2009)
6. Viswanathan, H.: Extending the Role of the Mobile Network Operator in M2M. In: 1st ETSI TC M2M Workshop, Sophia Antipolis (2010)
7. 3GPP TR 22.868: Study on Facilitating Machine to Machine Communication in 3GPP Systems (2007)
8. ETSI TR 102 732: Use Cases of M2M Applications for eHealth. Draft Standard (2010)
9. 3GPP TS 22.368: Service Requirements for Machine-Type Communications (MTC); Stage 1 (2011)
10. 3GPP TR 22.888: System Improvements for Machine-Type Communications (2010)
11. Holma, H., Toskala, A.: WCDMA for UMTS: HSPA evolution and LTE, 5th edn. Wiley & Sons Ltd, Chichester (2009)
12. Zhang, J., de la Roche, G.: Femtocells: Technologies and Deployment, 1st edn. John Wiley & Sons Ltd, Chichester (2009)
13. Tekelec: Towards a Personalized Mobile Experience: How Converged Subscriber Management Will Impact the Life of End-users. Tekelec white paper (2010)
14. Olsson, M., Shabnam, S., Rommer, S., Frid, L., Mulligan, C.: SAE and the Evolved Packet Core: Driving the Mobile Broadband Revolution. Academic Press, Oxford (2009)
15. ITU-T Recommendation E.164: The International Public Telecommunication Numbering Plan (2010)
16. Starsinic, M.: System Architecture Challenges in the Home M2M Network. In: Proceedings of the IEEE Long Island Systems Applications and Technology Conference, Farmingdale State College (2010)
17. Femto Forum Services SIG: Femto Services Version 1 API (2011)
18. 3GPP TR 22.368: Local IP Access & Selected IP Traffic Offload, LIPA-SIPTO (2010)

Developing a Real-Time Process Data Acquisition System for Automatic Process Measurement

Ye Zhang[1,2], Olli Martikainen[1,2], Petri Pulli[1], and Valeriy Naumov[1]

[1] Department of Information Processing Science, University of Oulu, Oulu, Finland
{petri.pulli,valeriy.naumov}@oulu.fi
[2] The Research Institute of the Finnish Economy (ETLA)
{ye.zhang,olli.martikainen}@etla.fi

Abstract. As the population aging is a global and unalterable trend, and the whole society is lacking of productive workforce to provide healthcare services, there is a pressure to develop smart services to support the elderly persons live a more independent life and improve the quality of open healthcare. This paper combines together the concepts of smart living environment and process management, we discuss a novel method called automatic process measurement that uses wireless technologies to collect process data for process mining and process analysis. Besides, this paper presents the real-time data acquisition system that is capable of measuring elderly people's behavior and nurse's behavior. We apply the system to three Linux-based platforms and evaluate it in laboratory and practical environment. The proposed system fulfills the measurement needs of collecting process data for automatic process modeling.

Keywords: Real-time data acquisition, automatic process measurement, process mining, Bluetooth.

1   Introduction

The aging of population has put severer challenges to the whole world, requires the concern and efforts of the whole society. We're facing the problems of lacking productive workforce such as nursing personnel to support the social healthcare and other services [6]. In order to create a more comfort, better and securer life for the elderly under this circumstance, a lot of studies on automatic elderly assistant systems have been conducted. This paper is a part of greater multidisciplinary research schemes: Value Creation in Smart Living Environment for Senior Citizen (VESC) project and "ICT, Service Innovations and Productivity" project. The objective of the VESC project is to support the elderly in their daily activities and improve the quality of open healthcare by developing technology-based smart services [1], the VESC project defines the future smart living environment for the elderly people, as shown in Fig. 1.

Contributions of this paper are that it combines together the concepts of smart living environment for senior citizen and process management, and proposes a novel method called automatic process measurement that uses wireless technologies to collect the process data for further process mining and process analysis.

M. Rautiainen et al. (Eds.): GPC 2011 Workshops, LNCS 7096, pp. 115–124, 2012.

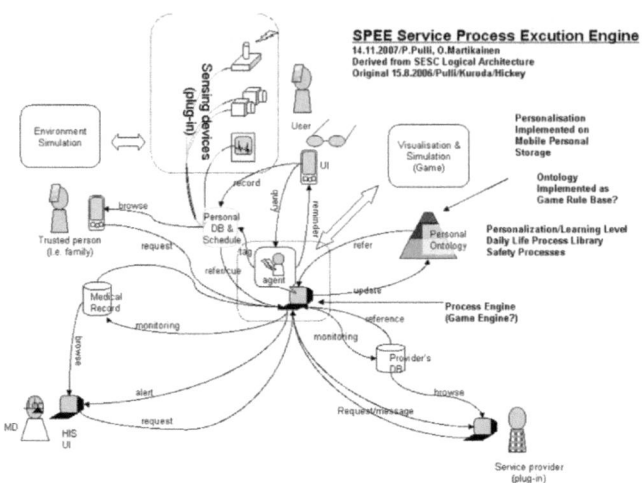

Fig. 1. The Smart Living Environment for the Elderly

In VESC project, there are need to study elderly people's daily behavior and measure the nursing personnel's behavior in the open healthcare process. So A precise model of the process is of paramount importance, which can efficiently presents the abstraction of the real open healthcare. Thus, it enables better understanding and systematic analysis of the process. Traditional process modeling methods usually use graphical modeling techniques, such as flowchart, functional flow block diagram and control flow diagram (CFD), in this paper we adopt the idea of mining process information from workflow logs [5]. Process mining technique extracts data from event logs and then generates process models automatically, those event logs are usually recorded by various information systems, as the main contribution in this paper, we design and implement a measurement system that is capable of collecting real-time process data and generating more accurate logs. The measurement system uses Bluetooth communication technology, it has the advantages of high anti-interference, worldwide license free radio band, low power consumption and low implementation cost.

The rest of this paper is structured as follows. Section 2 discusses related work. Section 3 depicts the measurement system in detail. Section 4 discusses the experimental results. Section 5 concludes this paper and presents the plan for future work.

2   Related Work

A great many studies on automatic elderly assistant systems have been conducted: in 1995, [4] conducted studies on learning the habits of old person and diagnose their behavior changes by using multi-sensor system and artificial neural networks; mobile robotic assistant systems, to remind old people about routine activities in their daily life, such as take medicine and eat, and to give them guidance in their surrounding environments as well [10]; real-time monitoring systems, [9] developed a real-time detection of the fall of the elderly by using tilt sensors and wireless communication technique; [6] developed an ultrasonic sensor network system that is used in nursing room to monitor elderly people; smart healthcare or home automation systems, for instance the B-Live home automation system that is implemented in 2007 by [11].

To a certain extent, those systems are much less intrusive and provide continuous real-time monitoring of the health condition of the elderly people. But, this is not sufficient, none of them considers to implement the measurement of nursing personnel's behavior in the open healthcare process, nor do they combine developing smart living environment with the concept of process management.

In process management, there are various of traditional process modeling approaches. However, they are time-consuming and require modelers with professional cognizance and the skill in process modeling. Models are defined by modelers manually, based on the analysis of process documents and consultations with process participators. This leads to problems, such as the individual experience of modelers and participators will greatly affect the objectivity of process models, large numbers of redundant data will influence the efficiency of traditional modeling methods [8], in many domains processes are evolving and people typically have an oversimplified an incorrect view of the actual processes [12]. So a new process modeling method called process mining become popular in recent years, the idea was advanced by [5] as early as in 1995, and was applied in process modeling field by [2] since 1998. Although this technique solves above problems in traditional process modeling approaches, it fails to achieve the accuracy of process data. It extracts information from event logs that are usually recorded by various information systems, so the data are not as accurate as real-time data.

3   Measurement System

Contemplating the background of VESC project, the expected terminal device should be portable and small-size, thus, we select two mobile platforms -- Maemo and Android. The system uses Bluetooth technology, and BlueZ Bluetooth protocol stack. The system records timestamps of activities by detecting real-time Bluetooth signal and distinguishing the global unique address of different Bluetooth devices.

3.1   Bluetooth Communication Technology

Bluetooth is a short-range wireless communication technology standard, using a worldwide and license free radio band -- Industrial, Scientific, and Medical band (ISM) at 2.4GHz. It has several advantages, such as high anti-interference, worldwide, low power consumption, and low implementation cost. Moreover, it supports transmitting voice and data simultaneously, and enables temporary ad hoc connections.

Bluetooth technology standard is for the inter-operation between various applications, remote devices should use the same protocol stack to inter-operate. Protocol stack is protocols that organized in a hierarchical structure, it is the core part of Bluetooth technology. The measurement system use BlueZ, the official Bluetooth protocol stack for Linux. Bluetooth capabilities of Maemo and Android platforms are both based on BlueZ, and BlueZ has been included in Linux kernel since version 2.4.6. BlueZ supports Bluetooth core layers and protocols, currently, BlueZ consists of many separate modules, such as Bluetooth kernel subsystem core, L2CAP kernel layers, RFCOMM, HCI, general Bluetooth and SDP libraries [3]. While developing the measurement system, we use a set of APIs provided by BlueZ to communicate with Kernel-level protocols.

3.2   Development Platforms

Maemo platform is based on Linux operating system (OS) kernel and many other open source components, such as Debian GNU and GNOME. It is a simplified version of Debian GNU/Linux, so with the help of Nokia Qt Software Development Kit (SDK), it is very easy to port the measurement system developed in any other Linux OSs.

Android platform is also based on Linux kernel, but actually, it runs on Google's own Java virtual machine Dalvik. Dalvik virtual machine is optimized for mobile devices, however, it's not possible to port Linux applications to Android platform directly. To develop the system for Android platform, Eclipse with Android Development Tools (ADT) plug-in are highly recommended, the biggest advantage of ADT is that it provides very simple ways to export signed/unsigned Android Package (APK). Another difference from Maemo/Linux OS is that Android platform use different Bluetooth APIs. In Maemo/Linux OS, Host Controller Interface (HCI) provides a set of unified APIs to access low-level Bluetooth while Android OS provides several classes to management Bluetooth functionality.

3.3   Architecture of the Measurement System

In the implementation of the measurement system, due to the difficulties to identify requirements completely at the beginning phase of our study, we use the iterative software development process combined with software prototyping approach. We firstly develop a prototype in Ubuntu linux platform with Qt Creator, a cross-platform integrated development environment (IDE), then customize it to mobile platforms.

The main requirements of the prototype are to collect real-time data and record accurate event logs. We determine the following data that are needed in automatic process measurement: who performs the activity, in our study environment, it could be a patient or a nurse; what is the activity, we use Bluetooth globally unique addresses to represent different activities; when does the activity begin and end, which will calculate the duration of an activity and analyze the sequence of activities, the system determines enter time or leave time by detecting real-time Bluetooth signals. Beside these basic data, further study can implement the acquisition of patient's real-time health information.

Figure 2 shows the boundary of the system and its use cases. User is the person who interacts with the system, and the system will record his/her activities. Bluetooth devices are set at different places to represent different activities, once the system enters the radio proximity of a remote Bluetooth device, a wireless ad hoc connection will be established between them [7]. Then, the system sends out discovering request and remote Bluetooth devices will response by sending back relevant information

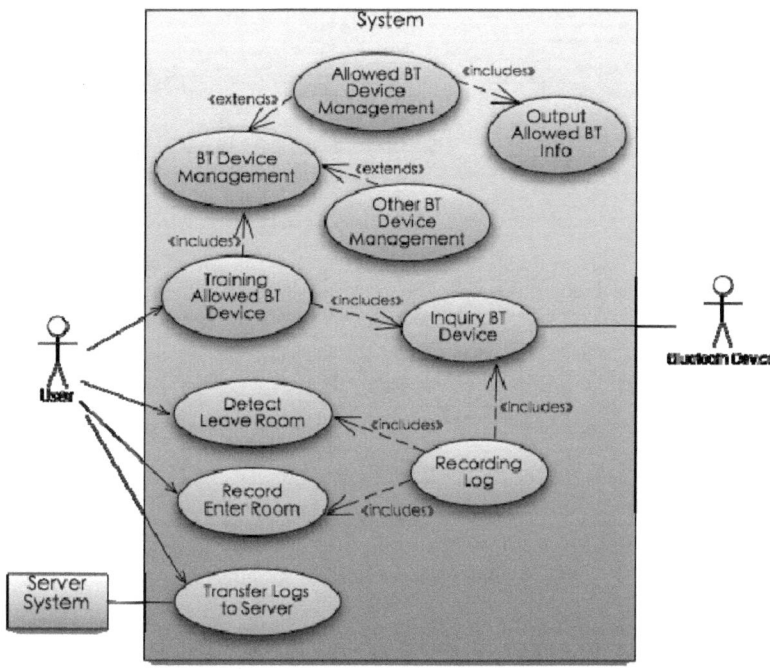

Fig. 2. Measurement System Boundary and Use Cases

(e.g. Bluetooth address, user-friendly name, device type, connection signal strength). The system includes three main use cases. First, an infinite loop of inquiring remote Bluetooth devices and process responses (see Inquiry BT Device use case in Fig. 2), it is the fundamental of the system. Second, Recording Log use case in Fig. 2, which collects real-time data, determines activity's timestamps, and creates accurate event logs according to the needs of automatic process measurement. Third, Training Allowed BT Device use case, it means to train the system to recognize which Bluetooth devices are allowed.

The architecture of the system is shown in Fig. 3, consists of four components, which are RTDAReceiver, BTDeviceCanvas, DevicesManaging and DeviceItem.

RTDAReceiver inherits from Activity class, runs in application's main thread, which creates a window that can present application's interface. It also responsible for interacting with users, managing local Bluetooth adapter and inquiring remote Bluetooth devices. It is aggregated by BroadcastReceiver class Intent class, IntentFilter class, and a self-defined ImageView class. Intent refers to the action to be performed, it acts as media typically: provides information for components calling each other, implements the decoupling between the caller and callee components. With IntentFilter class, the system can register actions dynamically, and only listen to interested actions. BTDeviceCanvas is a self-defined ImageView, it visualizes system's inquiring results.

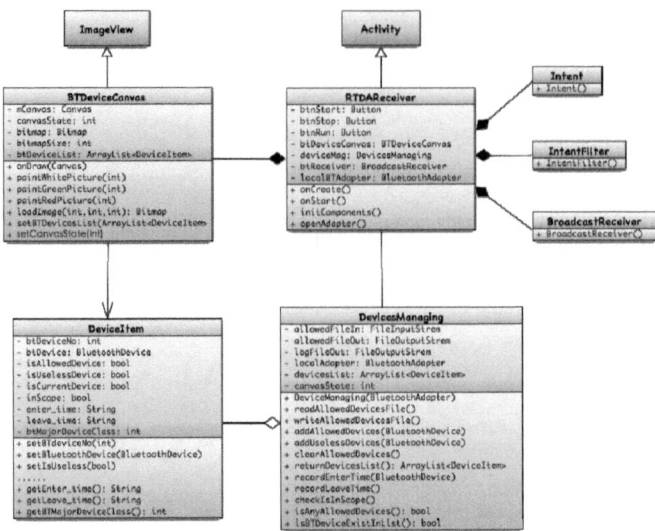

Fig. 3. Measurement System Architecture

DevicesManaging manages allowed Bluetooth devices, takes care of file I/O management, records relevant information of activities, including information of remote Bluetooth device, activity's begin time and end time. It has a DeviceItem type list, which saves Bluetooth related information (e.g. name, address, device class) and Boolean variables to help manage devices (e.g. is a device allowed or it is irrelevant, the number of allowed devices), and other variables to support the task of recording logs (e.g. check if a Bluetooth device is still in range, the enter time and the leave time).

3.4   User Interface

While the system stores activity records to the text log file, it visualizes the detecting results by painting them on a self-defined ImageView. The system takes the advantage of declarative way to build user interface -- using XML layout files, this separates user interface from business logic code completely, makes user interface replaceable. This design pattern is inspired by Web development (like HTML, XML files) that defines the user interface layout in readable structures, this facilitates the development and debugging.

The user interface layout takes hierarchy structure, two classes are used in user interface layout, View and ViewGroup. View objects are widgets and ViewGroup objects are layouts, each XML element has its corresponding java object. Figure 4 presents the user interfaces of the system, we design different icons to represent different types of Bluetooth devices, as shown in Fig. 4, mouse, PC/laptop, phone, or other Bluetooth devices. State one begins when the system is started, the system shows all in range Bluetooth devices (including allowed devices and irrelevant devices). User clicks Start button to trigger the system to change to training state, it will numbering all devices that are detected during this state, and stores them as

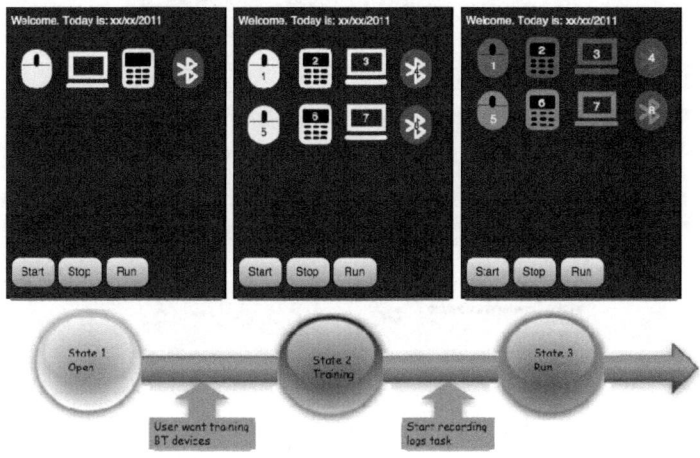

Fig. 4. Measurement System User Interfaces

allowed Bluetooth devices. User clicks Run button to start recording event logs, icon is green means that device is in system's detecting range, in contrast, red icon means the device is out of range.

4   Experimental Results

Three prototypes have been developed (see Table 1), and we evaluate the developed system both in laboratory testing and practical environment testing. Figure 5 presents the structure of testing setting, we use Bluetooth mice to simulate allowed Bluetooth sensors, also use other irrelevant Bluetooth devices like phones, PCs to support our testing. practical testing is conducted in Department 101 in the Helsinki University Central Hospital (HUS), the allocation of Bluetooth mice is shown in Fig. 6 (for example, Mouse 7 is in Room 3). We mapped Department 101 into a two-dimensional coordinate system for further analysis (see X-axis and Y-axis in Fig. 6).

Table 1. Developed Prototypes

	Prototype 1	Prototype 2	Prototype 3
Running Device	Mini-laptop	Mobile Phone	Mobile Phone
Running Platform	Ubuntu Netbook Edition	Maemo 5	Android 2.1
Development Tool	Qt Creator	Qt Creator; Nokia Qt SDK	Eclipse; ADT plug-in
Programming Language	C++	C++	Java

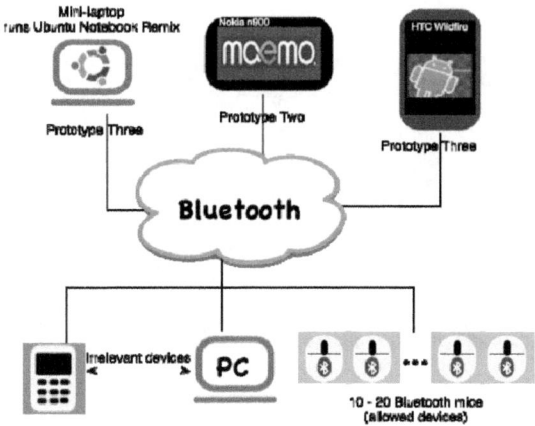

Fig. 5. Structure of Practical Testing

About 200 activity records were collected from the testing in HUS. In order to assess whether the workflow logs can be used in further automatic process mining, we plotted those records in the log files to make a line graph to show the nurse's movements between activities. Figure 7 shows the analysis results: the movements of the nurse in the testing, T-axis means timeline and P-axis shows the activity's position in the coordinate system in Fig. 6, red line represents the values on x-axis, blue line represents the values on y-axis. Based on this, we can conclude that activities that constitute a process can be clearly extract from the logs, the process data collected in the logs fulfill the needs of further automatic process modeling. But, for extracting process model from event logs is out of the scope of our research in this paper.

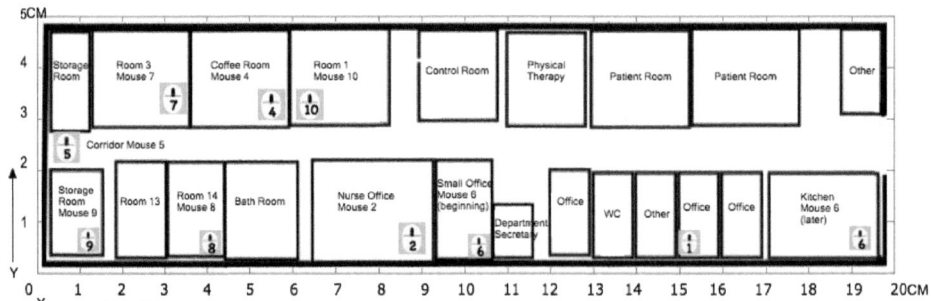

Fig. 6. The Map of Department 101 in HUS

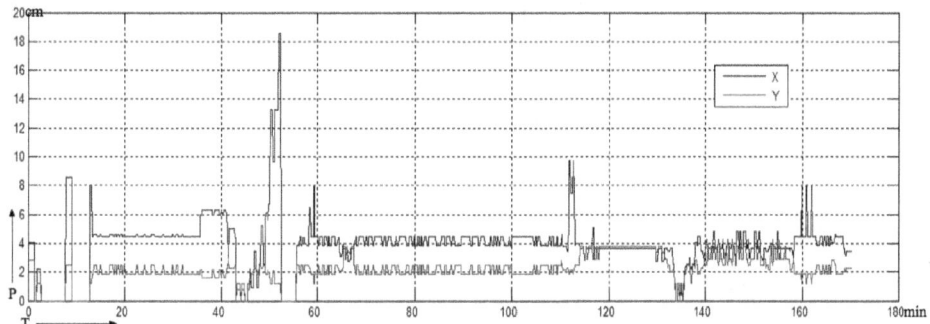

Fig. 7. Testing Result -- Movement of a Nurse

5   Conclusion and Future Work

We have combined together the concepts of smart living environment and process management. We have proposed the automatic process measurement method based on the idea of process mining. We have successfully applied Bluetooth technology in the developed system, which achieves collecting real-time process data for automatic process measurement. And We have evaluated the system in practical environment.

However, new problems and requirements are found during the experiment, our further research is to solve Bluetooth signal overlapping, and to improve the accuracy of process data. One feasible solution is to use Received Signal Strength Indication (RSSI) attribute of the Bluetooth ad hoc connection. Furthermore, we will support multiple sites measurement and multiple measurement devices.

Acknowledgments. We thank the "Academy of Finland MOTIVE/VESC" project for research questions formulating and research funding. We thank the 'ICT, Service Innovations and Productivity' project and funding from Technology Industries of Finland Centennial Foundation. We thank the Helsinki University Central Hospital and the Research Institute of the Finnish Economy (ETLA) for supporting practical environment testing.

References

[1]   Academy of Finland website (February 17, 2011),
        http://www.aka.fi/Tiedostot/Tiedostot/MOTIVE/
        Hankekuvaukset/vesc-conso.pdf
[2]   Agrawal, R., Gunopuloa, D., Leymann, F.: Mining Process Models from Workflow
        Logs. In: Proceeding of the 6th International Conference on Extending Database
        Technology, pp. 469–483 (1998)
[3]   Bluetooth Org: Bluetooth Specification Version 4.0, vol.0 (2010),
        http://www.Bluetooth.com

[4]   Chan, M., Hariton, C., Ringeard, P., Campo, E.: Smart house automation system for the elderly and the disabled. In: IEEE International Conference on Systems, Man and Cybernetics, Intelligent Systems for the 21st Century, vol. 2, pp. 1586–1589 (1995)

[5]   Cook, J.E., Wolf, A.L.: Automating Process Discovery through Event-data Analysis. In: Proceeding of the 17th International Conference on Software Engineering, pp. 73–82 (1995)

[6]   Hori, T., Nishida, Y., Aizawa, H., Murakami, S., Mizoguchi, H.: Sensor Network for Supporting Elderly Care Home. Proceedings of IEEE Sensors 27(24-27), 575–578 (2004)

[7]   Kansal, A.: Bluetooth Primer. Los Angeles: Red-M (2002)

[8]   Li, Y., Feng, Y.-q.: An Automatic Business Process Modeling Method Based on Markov Transition Matrix in BPM. In: International Conference on Management Science and Engineering, ICMSE 2006, pp. 46–51 (2006)

[9]   Noury, N.: A smart sensor for the remote follow up of activity and fall detection of the elderly. In: 2nd Annual International IEEE-EMB Special Topic Conference on Microtechnologies in Medicine & Biology, pp. 314–317 (2002)

[10] Pollack, M.E., Brown, L., Colbry, D., Orosz, C., Peintner, B., Ramakrishnan, S., Engberg, S., Matthews, J.T., Dubar-Jacob, J., McCarthy, C.E., Thrun, S., Montemerlo, M., Pineau, J., Roy, N.: Pearl: A mobile robotic assistance for the elderly. AAAI Technical Report WS-02-02 (2002)

[11] Santos, V., Bartolomeu, P., Fonseca, J., Mota, A.: B-Live A Home Automation System for Disabled and Elderly People. In: International Symposium on Industrial Embedded Systems, pp. 333–336 (2007)

[12] Van Der Aalst, W.M.P., Schonenberg, M.H., Song, M.: Time prediction based on process mining. Information Systems, Scopus 36(2), 450–475 (2011)

Adaptable Context-Aware Micro-architecture

Susanna Pantsar-Syväniemi

VTT Technical Research Centre of Finland, P.O. Box 1100,
FI-90571 Oulu, Finland
Susanna.Pantsar-Syvaniemi@vtt.fi

Abstract. A smart space can be any of our living environments which enrich our lives by relevant services and applications. With the help of context the smart space application can react to current situations or be proactive and take into account the coming circumstances. This paper describes the ongoing research how context-awareness is enabled for heterogeneous smart space applications. We report the results achieved i) of using context-aware agents for defining personalized views of shared information, ii) of a novel context-aware micro-architecture, and iii) of a new context ontology for the smart spaces, CO4SS. Finally, we aim to confirm that the context-aware micro-architecture (CAMA) with the CO4SS ontology is adaptable for multitude of smart space applications being based on different architecture styles.

1   Introduction

A focus of this research is on a smart space. That smart space is full of different kinds of objects, i.e. sensors, devices and systems interacting with each other in different techniques and ways. These objects can be manufactured to be able to communicate smoothly in the smart spaces. However, these objects can be existing devices and systems that are linked to be part of the smart space. The smart space can be e.g., i) a personal space built around a user and the user's device that will probably be a mobile phone; ii) a smart car; iii) a smart home shared with family and which has visiting friends and other persons like a window cleaner; iv) a smart city. The smart spaces vary a lot in the viewpoint of i) an amount on information produced and consumed in it, ii) a privacy of the smart space, and iii) a security and trustworthiness of information.

The recent state-of-the-art research results [1-6] point out an importance of a context-awareness; being context-aware will improve how software adapts to dynamic changes influenced by various factors during the operation of the software. They present that it is still challenging to reach the interoperable and secure applications that are multi-organizational, i.e. operate over organizational "boundaries". Many research items in this field are pointed out to be still open, including a distributed context management, a context-aware service modeling and engineering, context reasoning, a security, and privacy. In addition, heterogeneity of context information, an imperfection of context information, a complex mapping between raw context data (e.g., sensor readings) and abstract context information required by applications are

M. Rautiainen et al. (Eds.): GPC 2011 Workshops, LNCS 7096, pp. 125–132, 2012.

also open issues [7]. According to [1, 8], the effective design, implementation, and run-time support of smart applications are considered open challenges in the wide-scale pervasive environments.

2   Challenges in the Smart Space

The smart spaces are within reach. They need to have knowledge of the context. Thus, the smart spaces are obliged to be aware of their context. The most famous definition for the context is [9]: 'The context is any information that can be used to characterize the situation of an entity. An entity is a person, place, or object that is considered relevant to the interaction between the user and application, including the user and applications themselves.' According to the introduction above, there are still challenges to reach context-awareness in the smart space, i.e., in the people's environment that is enriched with smart functionality. Smart space applications are changing dynamically according to the objects and people interacting with it. The interaction in the smart space is based on the information which is challenging to model and manage because the information cannot be predefined and the information is heterogeneous. The information is evolving together with the various objects producing and consuming that information in the smart spaces. The objects can i) be manufactured by different vendors; ii) be based on different technologies; iii) follow the different standards; and iv) have different life cycles. To succeed with the smart spaces, we need to take into account also the existing, legacy, objects which need to be linked to be part of the smart space when it is reasonable. Hence, the heterogeneity of context information and the abstraction of raw context data, required by smart space applications, are our challenges in this research.

We see that the challenges mentioned above, need to be approached through three context dimensions: a changing state of an execution environment, an individual with own preferences and needs, and a context that is derived from the gathered information about who else can use or is using the space. Based on the literature, we claim that the derived context is not well defined nor well understood. The three context dimensions, similar to ours, are defined in the survey of context modeling and reasoning techniques [2]: a physical context, a computational context and a user context. That survey reports about the three approaches for the context modeling and reasoning: an object-role based model, a spatial model, and an ontology-based model. The object-role based approach has its strength in its support for various stages of the software engineering process. The weakness of the object-role based model is a 'flat' information model, i.e., all context types are represented as atomic facts. The survey reports that spatial context models are well suited for the context-aware applications that are mainly location-based, as are many mobile applications. The weakness in the spatial context model is the effort needed to gather and keep up to date the location data of the context information. According to that survey, the ontology-based model provides clear advantage both in terms of heterogeneity and interoperability. The user-friendly graphical tools make the design of ontological context models viable to developers that are not particularly familiar with description logics (DL). However, there is very little support for modeling temporal aspects in the ontologies. The main problem in the ontological model is that reasoning with, e.g., web ontology language with description logics (OWL-DL) creates serious performance issues.

We claim that the ontology-based model is the best way to deal with the challenge related to the heterogeneous context information and to reach interoperability between different objects in the smart spaces. A privacy protection of context information will need to utilize the specialized context-aware capabilities. We claim that the context-aware capabilities or agents need to be separated from the application logic to be able to offer generic solution that can be instantiated to be used e.g., for quality management at run-time. A survey about a context-aware service engineering [5] presents similar thoughts about the separation of context from the application. That survey classifies context-aware service engineering into two classes; language based approaches and model-driven approaches. The language based approaches like context-oriented programming and aspect-oriented programming follow the separation of concerns in which applications are kept context-free and context is handled as a first-class entity of the programming language while separate constructs are used to inject context-related behavior into the adaptable skeleton. Typically, the model-driven approaches introduce a metal-model enriched with context related artifacts, in order to support context-aware service engineering. Several model-driven approaches have emerged [5, 6].

3   Research Problem

The work to be done in this research aims to solve the challenges described above with generic context-aware micro-architecture [10] and the context ontology for smart spaces [11] that conforms to the context-aware micro-architecture. The micro-architecture refers to small software solution which enables the smart applications to be aware of their context and behave accordingly and even proactively. Based on the context ontology and the context-aware micro-architecture, we work to validate them and publish them as adaptable context-aware micro-architecture that can be instantiated for the multitude of heterogeneous architecture styles. Thus, the research problem is:

"Find a generic context-aware micro-architecture, which can be adapted to the heterogeneous smart spaces."

4   Research Approach

This research will be carried out within real and laboratory environments and because of that case studies will be used as the main research method. The case studies can involve either a single case or multiple cases, and numerous levels of analysis [12]. The case studies combine data collection methods such as interviews, questionnaires and observations. The evidence may be qualitative, quantitative, or both [12]. According to the guidelines introduced in [13], the case study is a suitable research methodology for software engineering research since it studies contemporary pheno-mena in its natural context. The research approach has the following activities, as illustrated in Figure 1.

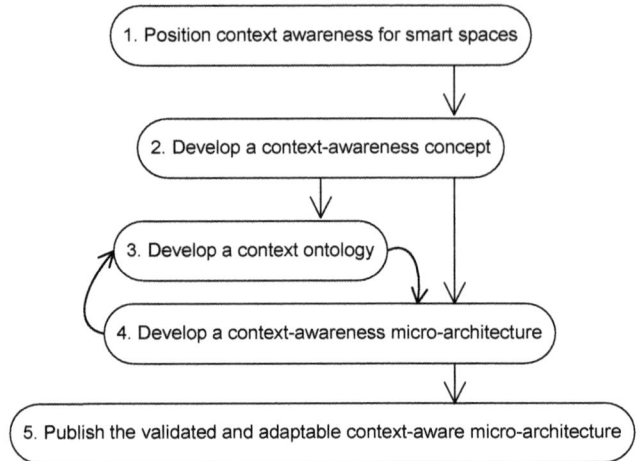

Fig. 1. Research approach

1. The first activity aims to do the state-of-the-art work and position the context awareness for the smart spaces. It will evaluate a relevancy of the common context definition in the smart spaces we are focusing on, more local than a global one. The use case approach will be used for positioning the need for the context-awareness in a Smart-M3 [14, 15] based software architecture with semantic information brokers (SIB), knowledge processors (KP) and smart space application protocol (SSAP). The position paper [16] was published based on this activity. We propose to shift the focus from the content to the purpose of context. Instead of trying to describe all possible types of context data that might be of interest for the generic smart space (SS) appli-cation, we assume that any piece of data, at a given time, might be context for a given application. Hence, we propose that 'A context defines the limit of information usage of a smart space application'.

2. The second activity will concentrate for capturing a set of new capabilities re-quired for achieving the context-awareness in the smart spaces. The aim is to sort out the relevant context dimensions by going through the different activities required for the context: acquirement, aggregation, interpretation, representation, and reasoning. Based on this activity, the novel context-awareness concept [17] was published with context monitoring, context reasoning and context-based adaptation agents. The con-text monitoring agent has been defined to be used for the security adaptation in the smart space application, as is reported in [18]. The first version of the novel context ontology is also formulated in this activity and we selected the ontology-based model

and a web ontology language (OWL) [19] for describing the context ontology. The reason for our selection is due to the OWL support for interoperability and heterogeneity that are needed for the ontology to be able to evolve in the future. The novel context ontology will exploit some parts from the SOUPA [20] and the upper context conceptualization [4]. The context can be used, e.g., 1) for adapting behavior of an application according to the available resources in the execution environment, user needs and preferences; and 2) for managing quality at run-time.

3. The third activity aims to develop a more detailed context ontology that supports the context-aware micro-architecture for the smart spaces. This activity tackles the context modeling challenge when context information is as heterogeneous as it is in the smart spaces. Based on this activity, the context ontology for smart spaces (CO4SS) [11] was developed incrementally and side by side with the context-aware micro-architecture.

4. The fourth activity will use the context-awareness concept as basis for the context-aware micro-architecture which will have software agents for the context monitoring, reasoning and context based adaptation. Based on this activity, was published the context-aware micro-architecture (CAMA) [10].

5. The fifth activity is for confirming and publishing the context-aware micro-architecture (CAMA) with the CO4SS ontology. The validation will be done by demonstration cases. This activity will confirm the context-aware micro-architecture and the CO4SS ontology and therefore solve the research problem of this research. We will adjust, if needed, the context-aware micro-architecture and the CO4SS ontology. We will publish the results of the validation cases, as is done in [21]. The adaptable context-aware micro-architecture is intended for instantiating smart space applications that are able to share understanding of the current and coming situations. This activity is enabler for the smart space applications to be developed and commercialized.

5   Research Outcomes

According to the activities described in the previous section, the outcomes of this research, as illustrated in Figure 2, have for the present been

1) The state-of-the art study relating to context-awareness and positioning of the need for provide support for context-awareness in the software architecture for the smart spaces [16];

2) The developed novel context-awareness concept for building up the needed support for context-awareness in the smart spaces [17];

3) The use of the context-awareness concept as basis for the context-aware micro-architecture [10] and for the CO4SS ontology [11];

4) The usage of the context monitoring agent for the security adaptation in the smart space application [18];

5) The case study were the context-aware micro-architecture and the context ontology has been used to create a context-aware application to supervise the process of the smart maintenance of the building [21].

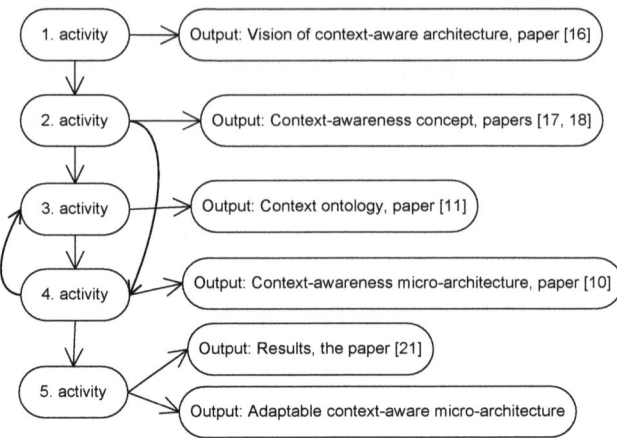

Fig. 2. Research outputs

The first results of this research are published in [16]: the context-aware middleware that extends the interoperability platform (IOP) of the Smart-M3 architecture by offering context-aware functionalities. We followed the separation of concerns principle by keeping the application logic free of the context. Thus, we positioned context-aware facilities to own entities separated from the context storage, SIB, and from the applications. More information about M3 framework can be read from [14] and Smart-M3 as an open source platform is available under open license [15]. The output of the second activity is the context-awareness concept [17] which consists of novel context ontology and agents for context monitoring, reasoning and context-based adaptation. That concept is based on the semantic context information triangle, as presented in [2]. Our conceptual context ontology is defined with three contextual levels: a physical context of environment, a digital context of environment and a situation context. Figure 3 presents the context-aware agents on the corresponding context levels. In [18] is presented the usage of the context monitoring agent for the security adaptation in the smart space application.

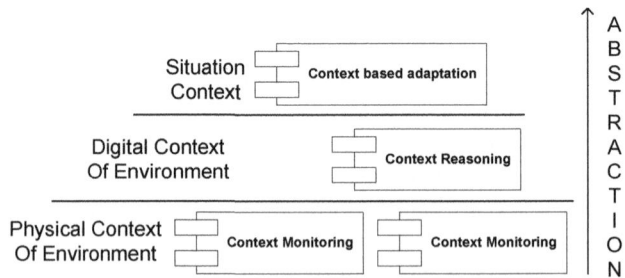

Fig. 3. Context-awareness agents on the corresponding context levels

The output from third activity is the context ontology (CO4SS) [11] which support the context-awareness concept for the smart spaces. The context ontology includes, e.g., context dimensions for the physical context of the environment, the digital context of the environment and the human context. The output from the fourth activity, the context-awareness micro-architecture, was published [10]. The context-awareness micro-architecture consists of three types of agents: the context monitoring, the context reasoning and the context-based adaptation agents. Figure 4 shows with the numbered connections the execution order of the context-awareness agents. Firstly, the context monitoring agent provides information to the semantic database (SIB) to be used by the context reasoning agent. Lastly, the context based adaptation is notified by the information upgraded by the context reasoning agent.

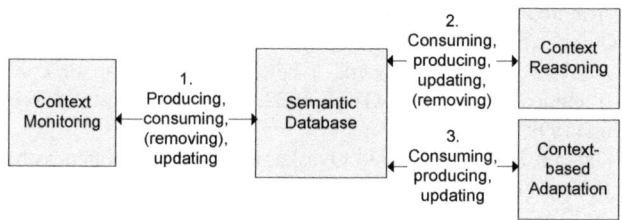

Fig. 4. Logical structure of the context-awareness micro-architecture [10]

Potential outcomes of this research relate to the fifth activity. Thus, this activity is ongoing what comes to the validation of the context-aware agents with the CO4SS ontology. We aim to validate both the CAMA and CO4SS in demonstrations where we will build smart space application for sharing information not only in one smart space but between different smart spaces. We plan to have demonstrations for the personal space, the indoor space, and the smart city. According to the validation results, we will modify the CO4SS ontology and the context-aware micro-architecture on need basis. The first output [21] from this activity presents validation of the context-awareness architecture by a smart maintenance scenario by implementing a context-aware supervision feature. In that validation case a generic context monitoring agent was used for collecting context information stored for the shared use of agents into a SIB. The fifth activity will solve the research problem of this research.

The potential output of this activity will be the published adaptable context-aware micro-architecture which will be one of the enablers for commercializing the smart space applications.

References

1. Hong, J., Suh, E., Kim, S.: Context-aware systems: A literature review and classification. Expert System with Applications 36(4), 8502–8509 (2009)
2. Bettini, C., Brdiczka, O., Henricksen, K., Indulska, J., Nicklas, D., Ranganathan, A., Riboni, D.: A survey of context modelling and reasoning techniques. Pervasive and Mobile Computing 6(2), 161–180 (2010)

3. Truong, H., Dustdar, S.: A survey on context-aware web service systems. International Journal of Web Information Systems 5(1), 5–31 (2009)
4. Soylu, A., De Causmaecker, P., Desmet, P.: Context and adaptivity in pervasive computing environments: Links with software engineering and ontological engineering. Journal of Software 4(9), 992–1013 (2009)
5. Kapitsaki, G.M., Prezerakos, G.N., Tselikas, N.D., Venieris, I.S.: Context-aware service engineering: A survey. The Journal of Systems and Software 82, 1285–1297 (2009)
6. Achillelos, A., Yang, K., Georgalas, N.: Context modelling and a context-aware framework for pervasive service creation: A model-driven approach. Pervasive and Mobile Computing 6(2), 281–296 (2010)
7. Indulska, J., Nicklas, D.: Introduction to the special issue on context modelling, reasoning and management. Pervasive and Mobile Computing 6(2), 159–160 (2010)
8. Smirnov, A.V., Shilov, N., Krizhanovsky, A., Lappetelainen, A., Oliver, I., Boldyrev, S.: Efficient distributed information management in smart spaces. In: ICDIM 2008, pp. 483–488. IEEE Computer Society, USA (2008)
9. Dey, A. K., Abowd, G. D.: Towards a better understanding of context and context-awareness. Technical Report GIT-GVU-99-22, Georgia Institute of Technology, College of Computing (1999)
10. Pantsar-Syväniemi, S., Kuusijärvi, J., Ovaska, E.: Context-Awareness Micro-Architecture for Smart Spaces. In: Riekki, J., Ylianttila, M., Guo, M. (eds.) GPC 2011. LNCS, vol. 6646, pp. 148–157. Springer, Heidelberg (2011)
11. Pantsar-Syväniemi, S., Kuusijärvi, J., Ovaska, E.: Supporting Situation-Awareness in Smart Spaces. In: Rautiainen, M. (ed.) GPC 2011 Workshops. LNCS, vol. 7096, pp. 14–23. Springer, Heidelberg (2011)
12. Yin, R.K.: Case study research: Design and methods, 2nd edn. Sage Publications (1994)
13. Runeson, P., Höst, M.: Guidelines for conducting and reporting case study research in software engineering. Empirical Software Engineering 14 (2009)
14. Lappeteläinen, A., Tuupola, J.-M., Palin, A., Eriksson, T.: Networked systems, services and information - The ultimate digital convergence. In: NoTA 2008, pp. 1–7 (2008)
15. Smart-M3, http://sourceforge.net/projects/smart-m3/
16. Toninelli, A., Pantsar-Syväniemi, S., Bellavista, P., Ovaska, E.: Supporting context awareness in smart environments: a scalable approach to information interoperability. In: M-MPAC 2010, session: short papers, Article No: 5. IFIP, USENIX, ACM (2009)
17. Pantsar-Syväniemi, S., Simula, K., Ovaska, E.: Context-awareness in smart spaces. In: SISS 2010, pp. 1023–1028. IEEE Press, New York (2010)
18. Evesti, A., Pantsar-Syväniemi, S.: Towards micro architecture for security adaption. In: MeSSA 2010, pp. 181–188. ACM (2010)
19. OWL, Web ontology language, http://www.w3.org/2004/OWL/
20. Chen, H., Finin, T., Joshi, A.: The SOUPA ontology for pervasive computing. Whitestein Series in Software Agent Technologies. Springer, Heidelberg (2005)
21. Pantsar-Syväniemi, S., Ovaska, E., Ferrari, S., Salmon Cinotti, T., Zamagni, G., Roffia, L., Mattarozzi, S., Nannini, V.: Case study: Context-aware supervision of a smart maintenance process. In: SISS 2011, pp. 309–314. IEEE Computer Society (2011)

Ubiquitous Framework for Creating and Evaluating Persuasive Applications and Games

Mika Oja and Jukka Riekki

Intelligent Systems Group and Infotech Oulu, University of Oulu, Oulu, Finland
`mika.oja@ee.oulu.fi`

Abstract. Until recently human-computer interaction has focused on creating efficient tools. However with the rise of ubiquitous computing, the focus is shifting towards applications that provide better user experiences. Persuasive computing has the goal of motivating people to live better lives. In this article, persuasive computing is approached through games and game design. There is an increasing interest in games, both commercially and in research. Applying game design to applications, gamification, and serious games are two different approaches to using games to motivate. This work is particularly interested in creating ubiquitous applications and games. I propose a framework that facilitates creation and evaluation of these systems. The framework provides tools for accessing measurement data, managing avatars and enabling ubiquitous accessibility. This framework is a step towards answering the larger question about creating gamification and serious games design in ubiquitous computing contexts. The feasibility of the framework will be tested as a part of this work by creating applications and games, and also by releasing the framework for third party developers.

Keywords: ubiquitous computing, human-computer interaction, motivation, software framework, game design.

1 Introduction

According to Mark Weiser's original vision for ubiquitous computing, the future brings computing from our desktops to the world all around us [1]. This can be perceived as something life-enhancing or something disturbingly invasive, and it all depends on the implementation as noted by Greenfield in [2]. As is discussed by Bannon in [3] the first generation of HCI (human-computer interaction) treated users as factors based on statistics without putting proper effort into understanding them. The second generation brought users into the equation and was mainly concerned with understanding how people work. Differences between this and the third generation are discussed in [4] by Bødker, and the third generation is largerly focused on experience and the home. The second generation created a lot of tools, but as Beaudouin-Lafon points out in

M. Rautiainen et al. (Eds.): GPC 2011 Workshops, LNCS 7096, pp. 133–140, 2012.
© Springer-Verlag Berlin Heidelberg 2012

[5] the WIMP (windows, icons, menus and pointer) paradigm of desktop computers has nevertheless stayed essentially the same since its first introduction in the Xerox Star [6], and new innovations have not been adopted into these tools. When discussing the role of interaction software tools, Myers et al. also note that these past tools are no longer sufficient for certain application domains [7].

If we consider the old saying "where there's a will, there's a way", it can be argued that the focus of HCI has been on improving the way. The assumption has been that there is a will, and moreover that the will is strong enough. This holds true in the work environment where the will is typically provided by a well-known incentive: salary. However, if we want to create systems that enable users to make the world better in other aspects of their lives, we need persuasive computing. This is the domain where user experience counts as people are free to choose how to spend their free time. The perspective of this work is to look at a domain where the will is greatly enhanced by applications: games. The idea of learning from games is not a new one - it was presented as early as the 80's by Malone in [8]. Since then, the idea has been presented in HCI research every now and then including [9] and [10]. Similarly, prototypes that use game-like features have been tested with users and found to be enjoyable (for example see [11], [12], [13]). It has also been shown that game-like features can motivate people to do tasks such as physical exercise [14] or generate interest in e.g. museum exhibits [15].

There's another reason to seriously think about games. In this day and age, people are playing games. A lot. To quote some numbers, a 2011 study by the Entertainment Software Association of the US consumer market[1] shows that games are played in 72 % of households. In Europe Strategy Analytics' European Digital Media Survey from 2008[2] shows that 71 % of broadband users play games. The role of games in the twenty-first century is explored by Chatfield in [16], providing compelling reasons why attention to games should be paid. McGonigal argues that gamers are escaping to virtual realities because reality fails to meet certain human needs, and suggests that we should seriously consider what kinds of games will be played in the future to employ the skills of these gamers in a world-saving context [17]. Reeves and Read present a rather thorough analysis of massively multiplayer online games and work, paying special attention to similarities between the two environments and requirements for the participants [18]. How should we proceed with making use of games and their design?

2   Related Work

As discussed in the previous section, Malone presented a set of heuristics that could be used to take inspiration from computer games [8]. He presents these heuristics in three categories: 1) challenge, including goals, performance feedback and uncertainty of outcome; 2) fantasy, including emotionally appealing fantasies

---

[1] http://www.theesa.com/facts/pdfs/ESA_EF_2011.pdf
[2] http://www.strategyanalytics.com/reports/ix7hx8in7j/single.htm

and metaphors; and 3) curiosity, including optimal level of informational complexity and providing well-formed knowledge structures. Dyck et al. introduce four design innovations based on their research of fourteen games [9]. They note that: games support the forming of communities, people learn to play by watching others, many games feature highly customizable interfaces and games use less interruptive means of communicating information. A broad discussion of using virtual worlds, with massively multiplayer online roleplaying games as the primary example, to make work more engaging is presented by Reeves and Read in [18]. The book presents examples how mechanics and dynamics from games can be used to make working more engaging. Likewise, Lin et al. discover in [14] that by creating a scoring system and visual feedback in the form of an aquarium and a fish users can be motivated to walk more and also to become more conscious of how much they exercise.

In third wave HCI, Bell et al. explore new sources of inspiration for designing for the home by defamiliarizing themselves from the modern home [19]. They explore the cultural history of American kitchen technology and ethnographies of English and Asian homes. In the article they present twelve statements that should be taken into consideration. Two of these statements are especially relevant: focusing on efficiency unnecessarily limits the design space, and the home should not be limited to efficient tasks and passive entertainment. In their discussion of ambiguity in [20], Gaver et al. present three types of ambiguity that can be considered useful. The authors also provide tactics for making use of ambiguity with the general goal of engaging the user more effectively when interacting with the design. In other words, the goal is largely the same as that of games, only the means are different. Aesthetic interaction discussed by Petersen et al. in [21] is in some ways similar. The key idea here is that aesthetics can reach beyond what is seen to the interaction itself. The authors propose adding aesthetics as a design element.

If we shift our attention back to games, there are two common approaches: serious games and gamification. Serious games are an old idea, and have been visible e.g. as educational games. According to Koster, the true power of games is learning [22]. People are hardwired to feel good when they learn new things - and games are excellent teachers. Usually they only teach things that are relevant within the game's context but they do so in an exemplary fashion [23]. The appeal of using this power to teach useful subjects (e.g. mathematics) is easily understandable. Gamification is a more recent trend, although its ideas are not exactly new. The working definition of gamification is "use of game design elements in non-game contexts" [24]. The definition explicitly excludes serious games, as serious games are complete games whereas gamification is a way of designing applications and services. Most existing gamification attempts follow the marketing strategies described in [25]: scores, leaderboards, levels, challenges, achievements and rewards. In recent years these techiniques have appeared especially on various web sites. Typical examples include user scores/levels, achievement badges and profile completition bars.

Existing gamified applications and serious games show that there is an audience. Nike+[3], a motivational platform for runners, uses feedback systems familiar from games, as well as user-created challenges, and has a community of over 2 million users. FourSquare[4] is another simple concept: when going out, players can do a check-in in a location using a mobile application and that way inform their friends where they are. The system uses points and badges, both basic gamification techniques, and has over 1 million users. One relatively recent example of a serious game is Foldit, a multiplayer online game, where players try to predict protein structures, that has produced useful results [26]. Another example is the ESP game, for creating image metadata [27], which has been licensed by Google for use in their Google Image Labeler.

3   Work Proposal

This work is mostly concerned with one particular class of applications: persuasive computing. In previous sections we have looked at both HCI and game design. There is a good reason to involve both HCI and games: ubiquity of computing is so much more involved in everyday life than, say, console games, that HCI must be involved in the design process, even when making games. The most fundamental difference between applications and games is that of the goal. Games have intrinsic goals that have been put in by the designer [28]. While this is not true for all games (The Sims for example has no overarching goals) it is true enough that it has been included in some definitions of 'a game' (see e.g. [28] for an analysis of several definitions). Tool applications have extrinsic goals that exist in the user's own context. Malone differentiates between toys (games) and tools (applications) in the same way [8]. He also suggests that using toy-like features in tools can make routine and boring goals more enjoyable.

If we consider this difference of goals, we can look at it from two perspectives which correspond to the approaches of gamification and serious games. In gamification, the task of reaching the goal is enhanced by game design to introduce motivating factors such as better feedback and subgoals. This approach retains the external goal of the task while setting sidegoals that aid the user in staying more engaged with the task. This approach has varying amounts of similarity with third wave HCI propositions discussed in the previous sections. In the serious games approach, the goal of the task is reached as a side effect of playing a game. The game creates a new goal, which is intrinsic to the game, and transforms the extrinsic goal into a consequence of play. The actual task is incorporated in the game's mechanics in such a way that it gets done. The designer is tasked with creating the rest of the mechanics in a way that produces a good playing experience. This approach actually transforms the problem into a pure game design problem where one mechanic of the game is fixed.

Neither approach is effortless. In gamification the big challenge is selecting powerful incentives that work in the desired context and have a lasting appeal.

---

[3] http://nikerunning.nike.com/nikeos/p/nikeplus/en_EMEA/
[4] https://foursquare.com/

In serious games, the problem is the same as with game design in general: creating a truly engaging, good game is really hard. If we look at persuasive computing, there are additional problems with showing that the system has the intended effect on motivation. Furthermore, because both of these approaches are in fact quite hard, can it be shown that they are actually worth the trouble, or could similar results be gained with easier methods such as simple performance visualization? In this work I propose to create a ubiquitous framework for making these persuasive applications and games. The purpose of this framework is to facilitate creation of applications of either approach, and provide efficient evaluation opportunities for developers. This work provides tools that especially researchers with more limited resources should find useful if they want to make these applications or games and evaluate their effectiveness.

The proposed framework is specifically aimed at applications that in one way or another encourage the user or player to perform a task. In the serious game approach, the approach is less nudging and more based on framing of the task. The platform provides the basic architecture for creating applications that have ubiquitous accessibility and make use of measurement data. The accessibility plan at the moment contains the use of mobile devices, desktop computers, public displays and RFID or NFC tags. Measurement data is handled with flexible plugin-based support for retrieving data from connected sources. The framework also provides the means to manage basic virtual world assets - avatars and their possessions - in a centralized way. Another important aspect that is included in the implementation plan of the framework, is evaluation support. The centralized approach facilitates extensive logging of user or player activity. The plan also includes constructing support for different means of doing ubiquitous computing system surveys (a good summary of techniques is provided in [29]), allowing developers to do surveys and researches to perform evaluation studies.

There already exist several platforms for pervasive and ubiquitous games that have fairly recently been built. Organizations participating in the IPerG (Integrated Project on Pervasive Gaming) [30] which run from 2004 to 2008 produced a set of tools for making pervasive and ubiquitous games. The UbiComp Solution package[5] by the Swedish Institute of Computer Science is most closely related to the work proposed in this paper. The package is built of Java libraries and facilitates creation of games that use small networked computers, sensors and actuators. Another academic example is the UbiqGames framework from the MIT STEP (Scheller Teacher Education Program) lab with focus on educational games [31]. There is also at least one commercial system by LocoMatrix[6], which uses smart phones and GPS for pervasive games. My proposed framework differs from these existing solutions by providing the important measurement data facilities as well as built-in support for data-based user avatars.

---

[5] http://iperg.sics.se/tech_space22.php
[6] http://www.locomatrix.co.uk/

4   Research Plan

The bigger research question related to this framework is the one from introduction: how should we proceed with making use of games and their design? What are the design considerations in ubiquitous persuasive applications and games? However, within the context of just one doctoral thesis, this question is too large. The purpose of my doctoral studies is to show that this framework is a useful step towards answering this bigger question. There are two key questions. The first one is whether the framework is found useful by other developers. One metric to evaluate this is to consider the number of games and applications made using this framework by others during the course of its development. More useful information about usefulness of this framework can be gained by using primarily qualitative research methods such as developer interviews and ethnographies. This information is not only valuable in showing the validity of the framework, but also to improve it and the development processes of ubiquitous games in general.

The second question is whether games and applications made using this framework have a notable effect on motivation. As discussed in the previous section, supporting evaluation of this topic is one of the design goals of the platform. This will be primarily tested by our own applications and games. The goal is to deploy these applications in the field and test them in real use. We are already planning first studies for an early application using this framework. In these first studies we are testing the feasibility and usability of the system in real use, and the effect of data visualization on motivation. The metrics in this study include user statistics and logs as well as qualitative surveys. In addition to providing good initial data about the framework in use, this and later studies will have a constructive impact on development of the framework. Furthermore, by analyzing the study itself, future studies can be improved based on the findings.

I have background in game design and development, and in the programming of networked applications for web, desktop and mobile platforms. During the course of this work, I intend to reinforce my knowledge in these fields, with a focus on serious games, pervasive games and ubiquitous computing systems. The work proposed in this article has already started, and a deployable test version of the core server exists and is capable of supporting data visualization applications. The next steps involve evaluating this test version for visualizing physical activity, and creating more user-friendly control interfaces for managing user profiles. After these basic visualization facilities have been completed, the support for plugging in application and game modules will be added to the core server. The exact working order will depend on what applications and games we decide to develop alongside with the framework.

5   Conclusions

In this article I have outlined a framework for creating ubiquitous persuasive applications and games. I have shown my motivation for building this framework: we need tools to efficiently create and evaluate these applications. Also the motivation for using games as a central theme in the framework design was explained: on the one hand, the motivational benefit of games has been shown; on the other hand, gamers form a large part of the population. Furthermore, the rise of gamification shows an increased interest in game-based solutions to motivating people. However it is not clear if these gamification attempts are a better fit for persuasive computing than serious games. I have discussed the difference between these approaches and also their problems in the persuasive domain. The framework proposed in this article is intended for implementing ubiquitous computing applications and games that use measurement data. The contribution of this work is the framework. In the course of this work, the framework's usefulness for developers will be assessed. This work is part of a bigger context about the design of persuasive applications and games, and the intention is to continue working with this problem after showing that the framework is a suitable platform for future studies.

Acknowledgements. The research work presented in this paper was done in the Devices and Interoperability Ecosystem - DIEM - project (part of the Finnish ICT SHOK program research projects). The project was financially supported by the Finnish Funding Agency for Technology and Innovation (TEKES).

References

1. Weiser, M.: Hot Topics-Ubiquitous Computing. Computer 26, 71–72 (1993)
2. Greenfield, A.: Everyware: The dawning age of ubiquitous computing. Peachpit Press, Berkeley (2006)
3. Bannon, L.: From human factors to human actors: the role of psychology and human-computer interaction studies in system design. In: Design at Work: Cooperative Design of Computer Systems. Lawrence Erlbaum Associates, Inc, Mahwah (1992)
4. Bødker, S.: When Second Wave HCI Meets Third Wave Challenges. In: Proceedings of the 4th Nordic Conference on Human-Computer Interaction: Changing Roles, pp. 1–8. ACM, New York (2006)
5. Beaudouin-Lafon, M.: Designing Interaction, Not Interfaces. In: Proceedings of the Working Conference on Advanced Visual Interfaces, pp. 15–22. ACM, New York (2004)
6. Smith, D.C., Irby, C., Kimball, R., et al.: Designing the Star User Interface (1982)
7. Myers, B., Hudson, S.E., Pausch, R.: Past, Present, and Future of User Interface Software Tools. ACM Trans.Comput.-Hum.Interact. 7, 3–28 (2000)
8. Malone, T.W.: Heuristics for Designing Enjoyable User Interfaces: Lessons from Computer Games. In: Proceedings of the 1982 Conference on Human Factors in Computing Systems, pp. 63–68. ACM, New York (1982)
9. Dyck, J., Pinelle, D., Brown, B., et al.: Learning from Games: HCI Design Innovations in Entertainment Software. In: Proceedings of Graphics Interface, pp. 237–246 (2003)
10. Jørgensen, A.H.: Marrying HCI/Usability and Computer Games: A Preliminary Look. In: Proceedings of the Third Nordic Conference on Human-Computer Interaction, pp. 393–396. ACM, New York (2004)
11. Ballagas, R.A., Kratz, S.G., Borchers, J., et al.: REXplorer: A Mobile, Pervasive Spell-Casting Game for Tourists. In: CHI 2007 Extended Abstracts on Human Factors in Computing Systems, pp. 1929–1934. ACM, New York (2007)

12. Chao, D.: Doom as an Interface for Process Management. In: Proceedings of the SIGCHI Conference on Human Factors in Computing Systems, pp. 152–157. ACM, New York (2001)
13. Chew, E., François, A., Liu, J., et al.: ESP: A Driving Interface for Expression Synthesis. In: Proceedings of the 2005 Conference on New Interfaces for Musical Expression, pp. 224–227. National University of Singapore, Singapore (2005)
14. Lin, J., Mamykina, L., Lindtner, S., et al.: Fish'n'Steps: Encouraging Physical Activity with an Interactive Computer Game. In: Dourish, P., Friday, A. (eds.) UbiComp 2006. LNCS, vol. 4206, pp. 261–278. Springer, Heidelberg (2006)
15. Schmalstieg, D., Wagner, D.: Experiences with Handheld Augmented Reality. Mixed and Augmented Reality. In: 6th IEEE and ACM International Symposium on ISMAR 2007, pp. 3–18 (2007)
16. Chatfield, T.: Fun Inc.: Why Gaming Will Dominate the Twenty-First Century. Pegasus Books (2005)
17. McGonigal, J.: Reality is Broken: Why Games Make Us Better and How They Can Change the World. Penguin, London (2011)
18. Reeves, B., Read, J.L.: Total Engagement: using games and virtual worlds to change the way people work and businesses compete. Harvard Business Press, Boston (2009)
19. Bell, G., Blythe, M., Sengers, P.: Making by Making Strange: Defamiliarization and the Design of Domestic Technologies. ACM Trans.Comput.-Hum.Interact. 12, 149–173 (2005)
20. Gaver, W.W., Beaver, J., Benford, S.: Ambiguity as a Resource for Design. In: Proceedings of the SIGCHI Conference on Human Factors in Computing Systems, pp. 233–240. ACM, New York (2003)
21. Petersen, M.G., Iversen, O.S., Krogh, P.G., et al.: Aesthetic Interaction: A Pragmatist's Aesthetics of Interactive Systems. In: Proceedings of the 5th Conference on Designing Interactive Systems: Processes, Practices, Methods, and Techniques, pp. 269–276. ACM, New York (2004)
22. Koster, R., Wright, W.: A theory of fun for game design. Paraglyph Press (2004)
23. Gee, J. P.: What Video Games Have to Teach Us About Learning and Literacy. Palgrave Macmillan (2004)
24. Deterding, S., Khaled, R., Nacke, L.E., et al.: Gamification: Toward a Definition. In: Proceedings of the 2011 Annual Conference Extended Abstracts on Human Factors in Computing Systems. ACM, New York (2011)
25. Zicherman, G., Linder, J.: Game-Based Marketing: Inspire Customer Loyalty Through Rewards, Challenges and Contests. Wiley, Hoboken (2010)
26. Cooper, S., Khatib, F., Treuille, A., et al.: Predicting Protein Structures with a Multiplayer Online Game. Nature 466, 756–760 (2010)
27. von Ahn, L., Dabbish, L.: Labeling Images with a Computer Game. In: CHI 2004 Proceedings of the SIGCHI Conference on Human Factors in Computing Systems, pp. 319–326. ACM, New York (2004)
28. Salen, K., Zimmerman, E.: Rules of play: Game design fundamentals. The MIT Press (2003)
29. Brush, A.J.: Ubiquitous Computing Field Studies. In: Krumm, J. (ed.) Ubiquitous Computing Fundamentals, pp. 161–202. CRC Press (2009)
30. Waern, A., Åkesson, K., Björk, S., et al.: IPerG Position Paper. In: Workshop on Gaming Applications in Pervasive Computing Environments, Second International Conference on Pervasive Computing: Pervasive 2004, Vienna, Austria (2004)
31. Ng, M.: UbiqGames: Casual, Educational, Multiplayer Games for Mobile and Desktop Platforms. Thesis of Master of Engineering in Electrical Engineering and Computer Science. Massachusetts Institute of Technology, Cambridge (2009)

Dynamic Data Processing Middleware
for Sensor Networks

Teemu Leppänen and Jukka Riekki

Intelligent Systems Group and Infotech Oulu,
University of Oulu, P.O. Box 4500, 90014 University of Oulu,
Oulu, Finland
{Teemu.Leppanen,Jukka.Riekki}@ee.oulu.fi

Abstract. Heterogeneous and resource-constrained sensors, computational and communication latencies, variable geospatial deployment and diversity of applications set challenges for sensor network middleware. RESTful architecture principles have been widely applied in middleware design. The new Computational REST architecture offers additional set of principles. In Computational REST, computations are seen as resources and interactions are conducted as computational exchanges. In this PhD thesis work, these principles are studied and elaborated further in the context of sensor network middleware. Middleware and system component prototypes are developed, evaluated and utilized by field trials in real-world settings. As a result, new knowledge is generated of ubiquitous sensor network middleware design and dynamically distributing data processing computational load in resource-constrained sensor networks.

Keywords: sensor networks, middleware, computational REST, web of things.

1   Introduction

Information and communication technology advancements accelerate the development and deployment of sensor networks, which are being utilized to collect, store and share information of different phenomena within environment and society today. Advantages of wireless sensor networks (WSN) over fixed sensor networks include dynamic deployment and changeable network topology [1]. Suitable platforms for heterogeneous sensor nodes include smart phones, PDAs, PCs, appliances in households, mobile data terminals and vehicle computing platforms. Also devices in public infrastructure, such as traffic signal poles, could be used as sensor node platforms. However, these devices have constrained resources in terms of computation, communication, memory, and battery life [1]. At the server side of the sensor networks, the sink nodes can be local or remote servers and even cloud computing platforms having virtually unlimited resources for data processing and storage.

Internet of Things interconnects everyday objects by using Internet protocols. The objects are sensors, devices and platforms, which then become Smart Things. Internet of Things applications then utilize propriety communication protocols layered on top

M. Rautiainen et al. (Eds.): GPC 2011 Workshops, LNCS 7096, pp. 141–147, 2012.

of Internet protocols such as TCP or UDP. The Web of Things has the advantage of using established Web standards with devices, which can have embedded Web servers running and integrate with any content from the Web [2]. The loosely-coupled nature of the Web and reusable common tools such as browsers, languages and interaction techniques can be applied to the real-world objects [2]. Along with the Web of Things, RESTful [3] architecture has been introduced and its principles are widely applied to the context of low-power WSN. RESTful architecture provides decentralized WSN with unified view of components, described for example in [2, 4]. Recent addition to the REST principles are the Computational REST (CREST) principles, suggested in [5]. The goals of CREST are the distribution of services away from the Web server and composition of higher-order services from established lower level services.

In our earlier research, we developed a sensor network middleware for traffic related sensor data collection and processing [6]. The system utilizes mobile phones with integrated sensors and external public services in Internet as data sources, using HTTP for data dissemination. This data is processed in real-time and results are visualized in an annotated map in a web browser. Moreover, we have developed a system for wireless monitoring of energy consumption of everyday electrical appliances in private households [7]. The wireless sensor nodes utilize 6LoWPAN protocol stack and HTTP for data dissemination to a centralized server, atop local IP-based panOU-LU WSN deployment. In the server, data can be visualized in a web browser and metrics of energy consumption are collected. Currently, we are advancing the pa-nOULU WSN by planning new sensors, such as environmental sensors, and implementing REST interfaces for data dissemination in the system, internally between services and sensors, and externally with client applications.

This PhD thesis work continues our work on sensor data processing middleware. Based on our earlier research [6, 7], we have identified the following topics requiring further research: enabling seamless collection and processing of data in the sensor nodes, utilization of multiple heterogeneous data sources, data dissemination and persistent data storage, efficient distributed data processing at different levels of services and in multiple stages, data processing capabilities conditional on the data type, and controlling and monitoring the system behavior. A related issue is the lifespan of data, from milliseconds to years, within the applications where data type, quality and quantity are variable [6]. Studying these topics helps to develop middleware that can disseminate data in real-time, has low computational latencies, has energy efficient components, persistent data storage mechanism and has sufficient privacy and security features. Also, in this developed middleware, loosely-coupled architecture follows from the heterogeneous sensors, variable geospatial deployment and diversity of applications.

The rest of this paper is organized as follows. In Chapter 2, related work is given, Chapter 3 presents the PhD thesis work in more detail and Chapter 4 presents the discussion.

2   Related Work

In the RESTful architecture [3], clients connect to servers to access resources. A resource is any component or information that needs to be used and addressed. Resources are identified with URIs in well-known identification scheme and should be available through uniform interface, such as HTTP. Here, simple HTTP operations are used: GET, PUT, POST and DELETE. Interactions must be stateless, so that all the information needed to fulfill request must be part of the request. Services can be utilized through hypermedia links in resources or service discovery can be made using discovery protocols, described for example in [2, 4]. "Smart Gateways" [2] in the sensor network can also provide composition of low-level services as a higher-level service and in addition can be used for abstracting a non-RESTful service. This is useful for sensors which don't have enough capabilities to run a Web server. REST offers several advantages over traditional approaches [2, 4]. Interfaces in REST are simple and uniform. Implementations are light-weight and easily scalable as components can be completely independent. Lastly, all features already in HTTP are available for use.

In CREST [5], computations are seen as resources and interactions are conducted as computational exchanges. Computational exchanges are carried out in the form of continuations. A continuation is representation of the execution state of a computation, even including the required data, in a way it can be later resumed. CREST offers several extensions to the architectural principles of REST: 1) resource is an abstraction of a computation and named by URL, 2) representation of a resource is a program, closure, continuation or binding environment plus the metadata describing it, 3) each interaction contains all information necessary to complete the request, 4) few primitive operations are always available but resource specific operations are allowed for creating new representations, and 5) presence of intermediates is promoted for use. CREST URLs follow the structure: //server/url_0/.../url_{n-1}/data/ and are not intended to be human readable. The interpretation of CREST URLs is up to the binding environment and URLs can be freely modified by intermediates. A single service can be exposed through a number of URLs offering multiple perspectives to the computation which can be even recursive. In [8], the CREST architectures are taken one step further. As CREST component peers can be seen as clients and servers simultaneously, the concept of layers in middleware could be replaced with symmetric computational exchanges. Layers and services are a matter of convenience, perspective and scope [8]. This could question the concept of layered middleware altogether.

A number of sensor network middleware has been proposed in literature. The Devices Profile for Web Services suggested in [9] offers service-oriented architecture (SOA) middleware for WSN's. Middleware components run RESTful or optimized web service functionality to interconnect sensor nodes. Nodes connect to the network by plug-and-play, announce their presence and offered services in the network and publish/subscribe events to communicate. However, the SOA implementations can be too heavy for resource-constrained devices and do not truly expose the Smart Things functionality to the Web [2]. Comparisons made in [10] suggest that RESTful web services outperform SOAP based approaches in both request completion times and power consumption. Another result is that when considering IPv6 addressing, request completion times in IPv6 are longer than in IPv4.

The DIGIHOME WSN middleware [4] for home monitoring systems supports REST interfaces for heterogeneous sensor nodes and computational entities, standard discovery and communication protocols, multiple resource representation formats and event-based reasoning. For the middleware, the authors introduce software connector encapsulation providing interactions between components, invocation, persistency and messaging. Component communication is event-based, events can be local or system-wide and event processors can trigger actions on nodes based situation changes. Default interaction protocol is HTTP because of its prevalence, also Web intermediates are used to modify data in transmission.

Recent example realizations of Web of Things were demonstrated in [2], where real-world devices with embedded HTTP servers, and Smart Gateways not supporting IP or HTTP, were implemented. Web mashups accessed the devices through RESTful interface, mapping the native requests, based on Bluetooth, for example, to URLs. The authors demonstrated mashup from the user interface in the computer to a physical device and mashup from a physical device to a device. Proxy servers were used for dynamically discovering mobile devices as sensor nodes and disseminating requests to them.

In the literature, other solutions have been described for these challenges. Sensor network can be "wired" for a task by configuration service or files. This wiring can also be routing or reasoning-based. For service discovery, protocols such as SLP, service discovery layers or agents can be used. For code migration, bytecode with virtual machines, migration agents or native code have been utilized. Possible data formats and representations include ASCII, JSON, HTML, XHTML, XML, binary encoded XML and even Java object serialization [2, 4, 10]. Built-in content negotiation feature in HTTP also simplifies the task of delivering data between components.

3   PhD Work

The objective of this PhD work is the development of scalable sensor network middleware and data processing architecture. The main features of the system will be 1) uniform interfaces for heterogeneous data sources and data dissemination between system components, 2) dynamic deployment of system components and 3) methods for distributing dynamically computational load in the sensor network. These features need to contribute towards energy efficiency. To achieve this, the granularity of system components needs to be studied: what are the component capabilities and what constraints sensors, data and services set in the system. Monitoring and dynamic controlling of the system will be studied, for example, by elaborating further the dynamic partitioning problem described in [11]. Tradeoffs between system features and requirements are inevitable, following from the variable device capabilities, system component configurations and diversity of applications. Another related open research question is the optimal number of sensors for an application.

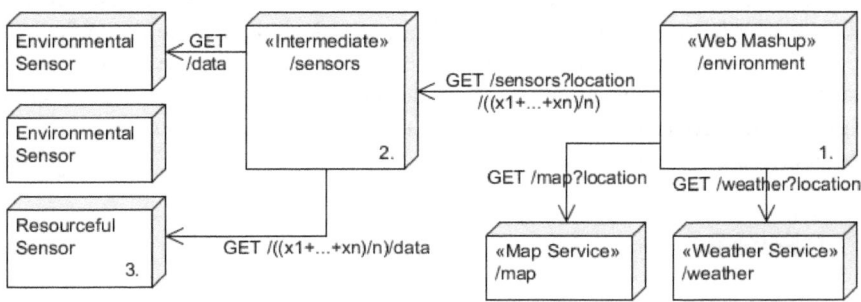

Fig. 1. An example CREST architecture for an environmental monitoring system

To the best of our knowledge, CREST has not yet been utilized in the context of sensor networks. In CREST, the origin server may not be responsible for all the computations as code migrates, thus the issue of computational latency is an important question. The system should have mechanisms such as concurrent processing and cost functions for minimizing the latency. One possible solution for this is the reuse of previously computed continuations [5]. To demonstrate how CREST can be applied in this work, a simple example architecture for an environmental service is sketched in Fig 1. Clients can access a Web mashup called /environment, integrating environmental sensor data with local weather data and visualizing it atop a map. An intermediate, called /sensors, is used to access the actual sensors. The mashup sends GET request with location parameters and a computation to the /sensors. This intermediate locates the corresponding sensor node and sends GET request to receive data from the node. Then the data is added to the URL, which is disseminated further to a resourceful sensor node for task completion (for calculating average in this case). When finished, computation results are returned to the mashup. In case this computation has already been partly computed, say weekly average till the previous day, a continuation can be used to reduce amount of required data and computational load. Also, the usage of intermediate is not required, but is used as an example to abstract sensors. In real-world, the intermediate could be for example a sink node or an edge router. The Web mashup /environment can itself be a continuation.

The middleware will be evaluated by having field trials in real life settings within the panOULU WSN and by using applications developed in research projects. In the evaluation, we are looking for answers to the following issues: 1) how much communication overhead is caused by the CREST principles and distributed processing, 2) are task or data query completion times reduced, 3) is the amount of data transferred in the network reduced and 4) can we reduce energy consumption in the resource-constrained parts of the network, such as sensor nodes. This work will be carried out in iterative manner based on literature reviews, implementation of middleware and component prototypes, tests and by collation of acquired experiences.

This PhD work generates new knowledge of ubiquitous sensor network middleware design and dynamic distribution of data processing load in resource-constrained sensor networks. Collected sensor data and processing results can be made available immediately as RESTful web services and new applications can be deployed to use since the infrastructure is ready. Possible applications in the system include promoting sustainable energy consumption in private homes, real-time traffic data services integrated with people's movements and other environmental issues in urban areas can be addressed.

4 Discussion

Expected benefits of utilizing CREST principles with sensor networks include: reusable data and computations in the form of continuations, efficient usage of resources with load balancing and distributed processing, easy context-switching and simplified deployment of tasks, services or resources to the network simultaneously promoting scalability [5]. Even service discovery mechanisms may not be needed at all in the system and it is possible to describe binding environments in the URL [8]. Concerning the given characteristics and requirements from Chapter 1, the proposed middleware is loosely-coupled and allows dynamic variable geospatial deployment of system components. How the code migration is actually implemented is an open question, but a number of techniques have been proposed in the literature. Heterogeneous sensors can be used, provided that proxies or intermediates are developed, especially for resource-constrained parts in the network. Constrained Application Protocol (CoAP) [12] could be one solution to realize this kind of system, being a web protocol optimized for constrained environments and having block transfer capability for larger amounts of payload in the messages [13]. For privacy and security issues, HTTP already provides basic mechanisms and these can be studied further. Interesting question is the role of the middleware which can be diminished altogether by these features, as suggested in [8].

However, REST is not perfect solution for sensor networks. According to [2], REST architectures are not very suitable for real-time information and event-based or streaming applications because of HTTP limitations. Computational latencies in REST and communication overhead caused by HTTP are inevitable issues that need to be studied. One example of such systems is the collection and analysis of traffic data provided by mobile devices, where real-time communication needs to be encapsulated with Web intermediate for higher-level services. Possible solution for this would be real-time "streaming channel" to/from the entities in traffic, controlled through REST interface operations and perhaps utilizing CoAP for data dissemination. It is currently unknown how data will be stored in the system for long term analysis, but this issue is also application-specific. Additionally, CREST URLs can be of size of ten's of megabytes [5], which is not very suitable for low-power resource-constrained sensor nodes. This could be one serious limitation in the system, but it can be addressed by using intermediates or proxies. To what extent CREST works with low-power sensor nodes remains an open question.

Based on previous research, the sensor network infrastructure in urban areas can be utilized to collect information and create new services in public and residential areas.

The middleware developed in this PhD work provides a platform for these services as well as contributes towards ubiquitous computing and Web of things.

Acknowledgements. This work is carried out in co-operation with Mediateam Oulu, University of Oulu. The authors would like to thank all the personnel in the RealUBI project. This work was funded by the Finnish Funding Agency for Technology and Innovation, the European Regional Development Fund, the City of Oulu and the Urban Interactions consortium.

References

1. Buratti, C., Conti, A., Dardari, D., Verdone, R.: An overview on wireless sensor networks technology and evolution. Sensors 9(9), 6869–6896 (2009)
2. Guinard, D., Trifa, V.: Towards the Web of Things: Web Mashups for Embedded Devices. In: WWW 2009 Workshop on Mashups, Enterprise Mashups and Lightweight Composition on the Web (2009)
3. Fielding, R.: Architectural styles and the design of network-based software architectures. Dissertation. University of California, Irvine (2000)
4. Romero, D., Hermosillo, G., Taherkordi, A., Nzekwa, R., Rouvoy, R., Eliassen, F.: RESTful Integration of Heterogeneous Devices in Pervasive Environments. In: 36th EUROMICRO Conference on Software Engineering and Advanced Applications, pp. 1–14 (2010)
5. Erenkrantz, J., Gorlick, M., Suryanarayana, G., Taylor, R.: From representations to computations: The evolution of web architectures. In: 6th Joint Meeting of the European Software Engineering Conference and the ACM SIGSOFT Symposium on The Foundations of Software Engineering, pp. 255–264. ACM, New York (2007)
6. Leppänen, T., Perttunen, M., Riekki, J., Kaipio, P.: Sensor Network Architecture for Co-operative Traffic Applications. In: 6th International Conference on Wireless and Mobile Communications, pp. 400–403 (2010)
7. Ojala, T., Närhi, P., Leppänen, T., Ylioja, J., Sasin, S., Shelby, Z.: UBI-AMI: Real-time metering of energy consumption at homes using multi-hop IP-based wireless sensor networks. In: Riekki, J., Ylianttila, M., Guo, M. (eds.) GPC 2011. LNCS, vol. 6646, pp. 274–284. Springer, Heidelberg (2011)
8. Gorlick, M., Erenkrantz, J., Taylor, R.: The Infrastructure of a Computational Web. Technical Report, University of California, Irvine (2010)
9. Abangar, H., Barnaghi, P., Moessner, K., Nnaemego, A., Balaskandan, K., Tafazoli, R.: A Service Oriented Middleware Architecture for Wireless Sensor Networks. In: Future Network & Mobile Summit (2010)
10. Yazar, D., Dunkels, A.: Efficient application integration in IP-based sensor networks. In: First ACM Workshop on Embedded Sensing Systems for Energy-Efficiency in Buildings, pp. 43–48. ACM, New York (2009)
11. Chun, B., Maniatis, P.: Dynamically partitioning applications between weak devices and clouds. In: First ACM Workshop on Mobile Cloud Computing & Services: Social Networks and Beyond, pp. 1–7. ACM, New York (2010)
12. Constrained Application Protocol,
    http://datatracker.ietf.org/doc/draft-ietf-core-coap/
13. Blockwise transfers in CoAP, http://datatracker.ietf.org/doc/draft-ietf-core-block/

Smart Spaces: A Metacognitive Approach

Ekaterina Gilman and Jukka Riekki

Intelligent Systems Group and Infotech Oulu
University of Oulu, Oulu, Finland
`firstname.secondname@ee.oulu.fi`

Abstract. Smart spaces provide services that support users in their daily lives. This requires the smart spaces to recognize the situations and adapt to them. Identifying the situation and adjustment to it in the physical environment has attracted lots of research, but recognition and adaptation at the meta-level has not been studied much. We refer with meta-level recognition and adaptation, that is, with metacognitive functionality, to evaluating the decisions made by the smart space and to adapting the decision making to maximize user experience. The main objective of this PhD work is to equip smart spaces with metacognitive functionality and the expected main contribution is a general framework for Metacognitive Smart Spaces (MSS).

Keywords: smart space, ubiquitous computing, metacognition, metareasoning, reasoning.

1 Introduction

Smart spaces are physical environments enriched with technology sensing the environment and changing its state. They interact with people in the environment, in order to provide them the right services at the right time, the right place, and the right situation. Smart spaces act as containers for different ubiquitous services and supply unobtrusive support for the user based on contextual information.

A lot of research has been carried out on different aspects of the development of ubiquitous systems. Context acquisition and data fusion techniques provide context data for users and applications. Research on context modeling has produced many formal representations of context, like ontologies. Context reasoning studies, in turn, have produced different approaches for deducing relevant information from context, such as case-based and rule-based reasoning. Many solutions to facilitate the development of ubiquitous systems by reusable middleware have been suggested. Also, human aspects of interaction with ubiquitous systems have attracted a lot of attention, such as how to address privacy and personalization, how to balance the ubiquitous systems autonomy and control, and how users can correct wrong system behavior.

However, not much research has been conducted on interaction at the smart space level. Instead, ubiquitous services and applications are mostly considered

M. Rautiainen et al. (Eds.): GPC 2011 Workshops, LNCS 7096, pp. 148–155, 2012.

in isolation from each other. Smart spaces are full of services interacting with users. Some services collaborate directly with each other, others influence each other without any intentional collaboration. Hence, good user experience requires considering the overall interaction provided by all these services together. As a consequence, the overall interaction cannot be tailored beforehand but must be considered at runtime.

Our research aims to improve the user experience of smart spaces. We propose to equip smart spaces with metacognitive functionality, which by means of self-analysis and self-regulation provide better user support. This is realized by monitoring of the execution of tasks and the overall interaction and adapting service functionality as required. The expected main contribution of this PhD work is a general framework for Metacognitive Smart Spaces (MSS). The results on metacognition research provide the theoretical framework [2]. We apply the metareasoning model presented in [3] to smart spaces.

The rest of the paper is organized as follows. Section 2 explores aspects of interaction in smart space. Section 3 introduces our metacognition approach. Research questions are formulated in section 4. We present related work with section 5. General discussion is provided in section 6.

2   Interaction in Smart Spaces

2.1   User-Smart Space Interaction

There are several aspects to consider about user-smart space interaction. First, ubiquitous computing spreads computing resources and functionality everywhere in the environment. Generally, there is no direct Human-System interaction. Interaction is always mediated through environment (Human-Environment-System). That is, human actions are perceived by the system through sensing the environment or explicit input, the system notifies users via environment as well, for instance by showing information on the displays. Hence, the environment itself becomes the user interface [4].

Second, as soon as the user is in the smart space, the personal borders of the services as the independent units are getting blurred. The interaction of the user with all services and devices of smart space are perceived by him as interaction with a single system [5].

Third, a lot of challenges arise when a user enters an unknown smart space, such as: How to advertise available services and their added value, achieved via services' interactions with the user? How to address personalization of these services, according to user preferences? A smart space should constantly learn user preferences from his actions and gradually target itself to match user interests better.

Fourth, several user and smart space contextual parameters affect the user-smart space interaction. Inexperienced user might need more guidance to use the smart space. When the user becomes more familiar, less explicit support from the smart space is needed. Moreover, user behavior can change in presence of other users, according to their familiarity, status, etc. User behavior is also strongly affected by the system performance, accuracy and relevancy of support. Hence, user-smart space interaction is always dynamic and volatile, evolving with experience.

2.2   Service Interactions in Smart Space

Smart spaces consist of many services and devices. Services directly or unintentionally (via a user or via changes in environment state) interact with each other to support users. Generally, from smart space's perspective, user support can be achieved both in decentralized and in a more centralized manner. In the first approach, each ubiquitous service of smart space adapts itself based on user and environmental context. That is, services are considered as autonomous agents acting in the environment. This approach introduces the following challenges: 1) Sophisticated techniques are required to achieve service collaboration, 2) Context acquisition can easily become overlapping and overwhelming, because many services can acquire user information to adapt their behavior, 3) Handling of conflicts, arising because of (un)intentional service interactions, and failures is difficult. In second, more centralized approach, smart spaces monitor the users and their interactions with environment (i.e. acquire context information) to tailor services composition to achieve better users support. This approach solves above issues, however it also introduces deployment challenges, issues of scalability, privacy and reliability.

2.3   Improving Interaction in Smart Space

Improvement of user-smart space interaction aims at providing better, more pleasant, trustworthy and reliable solutions for users' tasks, considering dynamic situations and user preferences. Serious challenge in this course is to measure the user satisfaction in unobtrusive fashion, e.g. perceived usefulness.

From another hand, we cannot improve user-smart space interaction if interaction between the services is poor. This issue leads towards autonomic computing systems design. Such systems are able to function by their own, without human intervention and posses self-* features, such as self-configuring, self-healing, self-protecting, and self-optimization.

In our opinion, to provide good user experience, smart space must be able to monitor, evaluate, and alter the decisions it makes, both from these decisions performance and user satisfaction perspective. That is, smart spaces should be able to do analysis of its own decisions based on the acquired information, evaluate whether user is satisfied with them, and modify its own decision making when necessary. In other words, smart spaces should possess metacognitive facilities, in similar way as humans do. We call such smart spaces Metacognitive Smart Spaces (MSS).

3   Metacognitive Approach

Metacognition research covers studies about reasoning about one's own thinking, memory and the executive process, controlling selection of the strategies and their processing allocation [2]. Figure 1 illustrates the general framework for the metacognitive facilities of smart space, applying the basic metareasoning model [3]. The physical space consists of users and devices that sense and act in the space, which includes different sensors, actuators and input/output devices(Ground level). This interaction can be explicit for the user, that is, he manually inputs commands to the input devices. Alternatively, this interaction can be implicit: the user's context is perceived with different sensors and other monitoring devices (perception inside the environment in Fig. 1). Services make decisions on what actions to perform to present information to the user or to change the state of the environment (i.e. what commands to send to devices) based on perceived context from sensor data and other available information. That is, the services perform reasoning (Object level). The commands executed by the devices and the actions of users change the state of the physical space (Ground level). Users act based on their own reasoning and also react to the devices' actions. This in turn, is perceived and triggers more reasoning and the cycle continues. Metareasoning, or more generally metacognition, builds a higher abstraction level to this model (Meta-level). That is, metareasoning is reasoning about this perception-reasoning-action cycle.

Metareasoning is analysis of how well the actions progress the tasks the services are performing and how well these tasks support users. It allows estimating and understanding what was happened, why it happened, and when it happened, why something went wrong, or why something achieved better results than expected, for example. Alternative strategies can be applied or even solutions can be created and evaluated to achieve the goals in dynamic settings. Metareasoning consists of both the meta-level control of computational activities and the introspective monitoring of reasoning [3]. Both these activities facilitate smart spaces to achieve better user support. Figure 1 makes it clear that Meta-level does not correct the actions themselves, but the reasoning process of the services. Moreover, Meta-level changes Object level, but not vice versa.

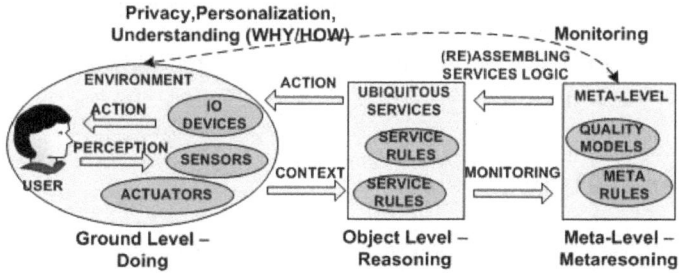

Fig. 1. The metacognitive approach

Meta-level of smart space is responsible for the following tasks: *Monitoring* of the system performance, state, possible conflict situations, and user satisfaction. Based on monitring, Meta-level evaluates how well the system (which in case of smart space would be the composite logic of services) supports the users, and creates an alternative solution for the problem if the system performs poorly. Monitoring also allows informing the user about execution, for example, justifying decisions and explaining failures.

Control. In our approach, control is building and modifying the services' reasoning processes, based on changing environmental context, user's goals and satisfaction and system performance. Control functionality is responsible for interpreting the collected data, evaluating it, and changing decision making when necessary. There are many challenges in building such functionality. First, models of good and bad performance in different circumstances are required (Quality models in Fig. 1). These models have volatile nature and they change with the system usage. Evaluation mechanism should be developed to judge the system performance and user satisfaction as poor or good based on these Quality models. Second, control mechanism, which actually changes the Object Level by constructing new or applying different decision making strategy, is needed.

We add the tasks of managing the *user privacy and preferences information*, which are not directly related to metacognition of the smart space itself and can be considered as a separate module of Meta-level. When a user acts in a smart space, a user profile is modified by a learning mechanism. This profile is used by the service logic assembling and execution mechanisms. Sensitivity of user-related information should be considered as well.

Metacognitive Smart Spaces are expected to support users in their tasks by monitoring task execution and planning, allocating, and tailoring the execution as necessary; according to user preferences, context information, and system performance. Metacognitive Smart Spaces define conflicts and failures and trigger decomposition of decision process in order to avoid them. Metacognitive Smart Spaces trigger learning when system performance or user satisfaction needs to be improved. Also, metacognitive facilities allow explaining the system behavior to end users. Generally, Metacognitive Smart Space resembles an adaptive system: It adapts its decision making process based on the contextual information, user satisfaction and overall system performance. Ideally, Metacognitive Smart Spaces should posses self-* properties of adaptive systems, such as self-awareness, self-monitoring, self-healing [6]. We emphasize the importance of estimating the quality and tailoring the decision-making process, that is why we call Metacognitive, rather than Adaptive.

4   Research Hypothesis

The purpose of this research work is to enrich smart spaces with metacognitive facilities. By doing so, we would like to evaluate whether interactions within smart space become more trustworthy and reliable.

General research hypothesis is the following: *Metacognitive Smart Space provides better user-system interaction support, by monitoring and tailoring itself according to its performance, context and user experience.* Better can mean faster, more pleasant, or reliable. We will address two sub-hypothesis: 1) Metacognitive Smart Space provides cause-and-effect relations details, hence users can improve understanding and control of the system. 2) We believe that the Meta-level of smart space can be realized using the same functional structures as the Object level. Our aim is to apply the rule-based approach in developing the Meta-level. We are planning to represent the Object level as a pool of rules. Rules will be applied also to make the evaluations and adaptations of the Object level of smart space (so called Meta-rules). The expected main contribution of this research work is a general framework for Metacognitive Smart Spaces.

Conducted research will be directed to prove outlined hypothesis and can be divided into three main phases: First, studying the theoretical issues, related to state of the art in smart spaces middleware development, adapting and autonomic systems development, and metareasoning aspects in context of smart spaces. Second, designing the general framework of Metacognitive Smart Space and building the prototype verifying the theoretical concepts. Third, development and implementation of the scenarios or conducting the simulation experiments to verify feasibility and usefulness of the approach, and incremental improvement of the framework based on the experience gained from the prototypes.

We expect that our research will help to improve the User - Smart Space interaction experience, user awareness and understanding of system facilities and, finally, overall user acceptance of the system, by providing metacognitive facilities for Smart Spaces.

5   Related Work

There is not much attention from the research community to metacognitive site of smart spaces. Mostly, existing research addresses separate aspects of smart spaces. McBurney et al. [1] explore personalization aspects of pervasive environments. Authors fairly note that instead of users, learning mechanism should be utilized to collect a user profile. Roman et al.[7] address meta-level issues at the application level in their Gaia metaoperating system. Their coordinator component manages the application composition and fault tolerance.

A lot of research has been done in monitoring of different aspects of information technologies, such as networks, software; however, not much studies were conducted regarding monitoring collaborating services for the smart spaces. Kang et al.[8] suggest USS (Ubiquitous Smart Space) Monitor, a monitoring system for a collaborative ubiquitous computing environment, providing monitoring and visualization of the collaborative applications. Lee et. al. [9] go further with their UMONS (Ubiquitous Monitoring System in Smart Space). It includes Analyzing module, which creates high-level, complex information via inference and recognizes system or application errors. Thus, this information constitutes initial levels of self-introspection.

Control of ubiquitous services is mainly focused with the logic adaptation or adjusting services compositions. White et al. [10] use context information to reconfigure services and resources to adapt the user access rights and protect user privacy. Xiang and Shi [11] propose to utilize personal service aggregation

(PSA) that maintains tasks, services, user's role, and underlying resources for each user. So the system reschedules the underlying resources, based on PSAs in case of resource collisions.

Nowadays the field of Autonomic Pervasive Computing emerges, which studies how key-main properties of autonomic computing, such as self-configuration, self-optimization, self-healing and self-protection can be achieved in pervasive computing [13],[14]. There are middleware proposals as well, e.g. [15]. Some of these considerations may help us in development of the Metacognitive Smart Spaces framework.

A lot of research were conducted about metacognition and metareasoning in computational Artificial Intelligence research [2],[3],[12]. Metareasoning approach has got a lot of interest for agent design [16], [17]. Cazenave [18] provides example of the meta-rules usage.

6   Discussion

Smart spaces provide unobtrusive ubiquitous user support. However, to achieve better user experience, smart spaces should possess metacognitive facilities, the same way as humans do, like "Is this algorithm sufficient to solve the task ? Or should I select another one?" Smart spaces definitely should include introspective monitoring and system execution control. That means, that smart space should be able to monitor all aspects of it: what is currently happening, are users satisfied with the decisions, etc. and alter the decision making process accordingly. Moreover, understanding of system execution quality is necessary, in order to achieve correct evaluation for tailoring. For instance, if a user is not satisfied with the efficiency of the service, a system should find out another algorithm or migrate execution on more powerful devices.

We are assured that some sorts of metacognitive facilities are necessary to achieve better user experience in smart spaces, hence this work is important. This research is at the early stage and our main interests are on the required control mechanisms of Metacognitive Smart Space.

References

1. McBurney, S., Papadopoulou, E., Taylor, N., Williams, H.: Adapting Pervasive Environments through Machine Learning and Dynamic Personalization. In: International Symposium on Parallel and Distributed Processing with Applications, pp. 395–402. IEEE Computer Society, Los Alamitos (2008)
2. Cox, M.: Metacognition in computation: A selected research review. Artif. Intell. 169(2), 104–141 (2005)
3. Cox, M., Raja, A.: Metareasoning: a manifesto. In: Metareasoning: Thinking about Thinking workshop held within 23 AAAI Conference on Artificial Intelligence (2008)
4. Schmidt, A., Kranz, M., Holleis, P.: Interacting with the ubiquitous computer: towards embedding interaction. In: The 2005 Joint Conference on Smart Objects and Ambient Intelligence: Innovative Context-Aware Services: Usages and Technologies (sOc-EUSAI 2005), pp. 147–152. ACM, New York (2005)

5. Wu, C.-L., Fu, L.-C.: Analysis and evaluation of system integration models for human-system interaction in UbiComp environments. In: The 2nd Conference on Human System Interactions, pp. 672–678. IEEE Computer Society, Washington (2009)
6. Salehie, M., Tahvildari, L.: Self-adaptive software: Landscape and research challenges. ACM Trans. Auton. Adapt. Syst. 4(2), Article 14, 42 pages (2009)
7. Roman, M., Hess, C., Cerqueira, R., Ranganathan, A., Campbell, R.H., Nahrstedt, K.: A Middleware Infrastructure for Active Spaces. IEEE Pervas. Comput. 1(4), 74–83 (2002)
8. Kang, K., Song, J., Kim, J., Park, H., Cho, W.-D.: USS Monitor: A Monitoring System for Collaborative Ubiquitous Computing Environment. IEEE T. Consum. Electr. 53(3), 911–916 (2007)
9. Lee, H.-N., Lim, S.-H., Kim, J.-H.: UMONS: Ubiquitous monitoring system in smart space. IEEE T. Consum. Electr. 55(3), 1056–1064 (2009)
10. White, M., Jennings, B., Osmani, V., van der Meer, S.: Context driven, user-centric access control for smart spaces. In: The IEE International Workshop on Intelligent Environments, pp. 13–19. Institution of Electrical Engineers, London (2005)
11. Xiang, P., Shi, Y.C.: Resource management based on personal service aggregations in smart spaces. In: Third IEEE Workshop on Software Technologies for Future Embedded and Ubiquitous Systems, pp. 39–42. IEEE Computer Society, Los Alamitos (2005)
12. Anderson, M.L., Oates, T.: A Review of Recent Research in Metareasoning and Metalearning. AI Magazine 28(1), 7–16 (2007)
13. Gouin-Vallerand, C., Abdulrazak, B., Giroux, S., Mokhtari, M.: Toward autonomic pervasive computing. In: Tenth International Conference on Information Integration and Web-based Applications and Services, pp. 673–676. ACM, New York (2008)
14. Ahmed, S., Ahmed, S.I., Sharmin, M., Hasan, C.S.: Self-healing for autonomic pervasive computing. In: Vasilakos, A.V., Parashar, M., Karnouskos, S., Pedrycz, W. (eds.) Autonomic Communication, pp. 285–305. Springer, Heidelberg (2009)
15. Trumler, W., Petzold, J., Bagci, F., Ungerer, T.: AMUN - autonomic middleware for ubiquitous environments applied to the smart doorplate project. In: International Conference on Autonomic Computing, pp. 274–275. IEEE Computer Society, Los Alamitos (2004)
16. Raja, A., Lesser, V.: Coordinating Agents' Meta-level Control. In: AAAI 2008 Workshop on Metareasoning: Thinking about Thinking. AAAI Press (2008)
17. Kennedy, C.M.: Decentralized metacognition in context-aware autonomous systems: some key challenges. In: AAAI 2010 Workshop on Metacognition for Robust Social Systems (2010)
18. Cazenave, T.: Metarules to improve tactical Go knowledge. Inf. Sci. Inf. Comput. Sci. 154(3-4), 173–188 (2003)

A Conceptual Framework
for Enabling Community-Driven Extensible, Open
and Privacy-Preserving Ubiquitous Computing Networks

Tomas Lindén

MediaTeam Oulu, Department of Electrical and Information Engineering
P.O. Box 4500, 90014 University of Oulu, Finland
firstname.lastname@ee.oulu.fi

Abstract. Ubiquitous computing is quickly becoming mainstream technology and one "killer app" in the field is that it makes unprecedented amounts of data available for data mining purposes. Advanced knowledge discovery techniques make it possible to create detailed profiles of individuals by combining and enriching data collected from a variety of different anonymous data sources. Access to this kind of data may itself become a key driving factor of large-scale ubiquitous computing deployment efforts in the future. Here, a proposal for a set of criteria and enabling technologies for creating low-cost, privacy-preserving grassroots-driven ubiquitous computing applications and infrastructures is outlined. Further, it is argued that a empowered community dedicated to the creation of a privacy-preserving ubiquitous computing ecology might act as a strong-enough counter-force against large-scale industrial deployments that intend to capitalize on this emerging, and potentially fertile market. Additionally, some early results from a real-life deployment of a network of public displays, which implements some of these principles, is also presented.

Keywords: Ubiquitous computing, privacy, community-driven computing.

1   Introduction

The ubiquitous computing revolution, as envisioned by Mark Weiser two decades ago, has already begun. One of the areas where the transformation is currently underway is the public spaces, where a variety of ICT-equipment is increasingly being deployed. These include different kinds of wireless data connectivity, such as free-to-use wireless LANs, Bluetooth access points and high-speed cellular networks, various kinds of public displays, including digital signage screens and information kiosks, as well as a multitude of sensors, such as different kinds of cameras and weather and air pollution stations.

This arena, where urban computing test-beds are now being setup, may be perceived as a playground for big players only, such as big-name street marketers, large mobile phone and internet operators and various surveillance firms – a field to

M. Rautiainen et al. (Eds.): GPC 2011 Workshops, LNCS 7096, pp. 156–163, 2012.

which ordinary citizens do not currently have easy access, due to the high initial costs involved when deploying novel applications in new application domains.

These early players are getting a head-start in the race for gaining a foothold in the new world that the ubiquitous computing transformation will result in. This, in combination with the large amounts of data these new infrastructures are increasingly generating on the daily activities of people, may as a side-effect, become a threat to our privacy [1], and indirectly, to our courage to wield our right to free speech [2].

The author's hypothesis is that, if people were knowledgeable enough regarding the risks of privacy deterioration, and if they were given easy enough access to building their own privacy-preserving ubiquitous computing networks, then enough counter-force might be built and hopefully reverse the already ongoing privacy deterioration process.

In this doctoral colloquium paper, a proposal of key factors needed for enabling a community-driven approach for building a privacy-preserving and grassroots-empowering ubiquitous computing ecosystem is outlined. As an example of how these concepts might be realized technology-wise, a practical, field-tested solution for building extensible and open public display networks using Web and hypervisor technology is also briefly presented. The approach, as outlined here, draws upon a variety of previous work from different fields, with the end-result being novel to the author's knowledge.

The rest of this paper is structured as follows. First, in chapter 2, the problem domain that this paper addresses is discussed. Then, in chapter 3, we outline the key components of a community-based solution that might address the problems. In chapter 4 the methodological approach for the author's thesis work is briefly outlined, in chapter 5 the progress in the thesis work so far is described, and finally, in chapter 6, why these results are significant to the field of ubiquitous computing.

2   The Privacy Problem in Ubiquitous Computing

Our lives are already being recorded to a large degree with data from a wide variety of sources, such as mobile phone positioning data, customer loyalty card swipes, internet operator traffic logs, and online advertiser's IP-tracking traces, resulting in information on where we are, what we do and who we interact with increasingly being stored in large databases. Once the ubiquitous computing revolution matures, we will be surrounded by thousands of small, wireless computers constantly recording and forwarding pieces of data [3] – which will cause an explosion in the amounts of information becoming available for gathering, storage and subsequent analysis.

By consolidating data, originating from different sources, and using data mining association rules, it becomes possible to infer new pieces of information that are not explicitly present in the original data sets [4]. Techniques, like pattern or subject-based data mining, originally developed for finding vague patterns of terrorist activity in large amounts of data [5], can equally well be used for building profiles of ordinary people. This becomes a potential problem if a person's approval has somehow been acquired, such as via some free cloud computing service's terms of service contract, to augment his or hers profile with information obtained elsewhere or through other means, such as data mining. Further, this provides a way to circumvent legislative restrictions that would otherwise prevent such data inferring or associations from being performed. Additionally, people are more willing to give out information about them when they are not explicitly "logged in" [6]. Given the observations above, people may act under a false impression of anonymity, thus enabling more data to be collected and associated with them without them being aware of it.

A database's value grows as the amount and variety of data stored in it increases, since data mining techniques assumingly become more effective at finding weak patterns when there is more data to work with. With increased value, also the risks of data theft and abuse increase.

There are technical ways of reducing risks of sensitive data leaking out of a database [7], but they do not give complete protection, especially if a database is compromised. These are problems people should be aware of, and when educated about these kinds of risks, people tend to be less willing to subject themselves to them [6].

Another, more subtle, problem associated with privacy deterioration is that once people become aware of their lack of privacy, the risks it implies, and if they feel powerless to do something about it, then there is a further risk of damaging people's sense of their right to free speech as well. [2] The rationale behind this is that if a person feels monitored and feels that an activity that is to be undertaken might seem suspicious and subsequently used in a harmful way against the individual, then one might subconsciously start to inhibit one's actions in order to reduce the risk of others getting hold of potentially harmful pieces of evidence. This sense of being monitored undermines creativity in a subtle way. Additionally, once a piece of data has been collected, it is hard to completely erase because it is not always clear exactly where copies of it are being stored. As an example, privacy policies for online services often exempt erasing of personal data from backup copies, for plausible convenience reasons on the database operator's part, even if a person has the right to have it erased from the main repository.

Therefore, in the light of the potential of misuse when concentrating large amounts of personal data, and people's general unwillingness to give up their privacy when they achieve enough awareness, the author suggests we should, from the onset, try to put in preventive measures for non-constructive data collection from happening. Since information is power, once the ubiquitous computing becomes established in our society, backtracking becomes harder, because of the various data-centric value networks that will at that point have become established.

3   Enabling Community-Driven, Extensible, Open and Privacy-Preserving Ubiquitous Computing

"Privacy is the claim of individuals, groups, or institutions to determine for themselves when, how, and to what extent information about them is communicated to others." --Westin, A.F., Privacy and Freedom. New York NY: Atheneum, 1967.

The key point of the author's thesis is to come up with practical ways of ensuring that data stays with those whom it pertains to, that is the people themselves and is disseminated only in a controlled fashion and then only with full knowledge of its implications. Hypothetically, this might be achieved if people were:

A) Aware of today's and upcoming potential threats to their privacy and the implications of giving in to embracing privacy-compromised technology.

B) Given compelling, privacy-preserving technological alternatives.

In order to increase the chances of these alternatives to be effective privacy-wise and actually be of interest to anyone to any significant degree, they would have to satisfy certain criteria in order to increases their attractiveness. A proposal of such factors is listed below. This list is by no means meant to be exhaustive, only to serve as a starting point for further discussion. These alternatives should be:

1. *Trustworthy*: There should be a mechanism for privacy-certifying hardware and software and it should be easy to verify that already deployed equipment and software truly are what they appear to be. In case of violation, certificates should also be easy to revoke.

2. *Affordable*: Compatible hardware should be low-cost and easy to come by (that is, be based on commodity hardware) as well as easy to deploy and maintain.

3. *Open*: Compatible software should be easy to create, share, install, configure, update, and interoperate.

4. *Resilient*: These alternative ubiquitous computing devices, infrastructures and applications should exhibit high resilience with regard to service disruptions, such as naturally occurring faults (e.g. network problems), deliberate attacks (e.g. denial-of-service attacks) and take-downs (e.g. through legal means).

A set of concepts and technologies which, taken together, might satisfy the criteria above, are listed below. A proof-of-concept implementation is also being built that incorporates many of these principles, which is discussed further in chapter 5.

i. *Hardware virtualization* and *software appliances:* Harmonizes heterogeneous hardware and makes it possible to build a hardware-agnostic, common software platform that enables software development across a wide variety of devices. A software appliance is a self-contained piece of software, packaged along with an operating system, which can be installed either directly, on bare-metal hardware, or on top of a hypervisor.

ii. *Web technology:* The Web technologies have large, established developer and code bases and Web programming has a relatively low learning curve. The Web supports building both rich, graphical applications as well as machine-to-machine interfaces (i.e. Web services). They form a corner-stone of the proposed community-driven application development, but other application development techniques should be supported in addition.

iii. *Fair information principles:* These are a collection of privacy-preserving principles, eight in total, drawn up by the Organization for Economic Cooperation and Development in 1980 [1]. They form a starting point, which could be used for building an assessment framework, against which ubiquitous computing applications could be compared to, with regard to privacy preservation.

iv.   *Open code review, code signing* and *privacy certificates:* Code signing (and the resulting certificate) enables making sure that a piece of software has not been tampered with after the certificate was issued. Ideally, the authority that issues the certificate employs an open code review process, which makes it possible for external parties to later check on which grounds a privacy certificate was issued (such as against the free information principles, above).

v.   *Trusted computing:* Ensures that the device's software platform and underlying hypervisor/hardware has not been tampered with by verifying the Trusted Platform Module's (TPM) integrity and authenticity. Potentially makes it possible to verify that privacy-certified applications run on privacy-vise safe equipment and do not contain any hidden eavesdropping components. It is important that the TPM is only used for verifying that the underlying hardware and hypervisor is intact, since the TPM may also contain notification channels, such as for digital rights management purposes, and thus be privacy-compromising by itself [8].

vi.   *Free software*: A liberal type of open source software that can freely, or with only minimal restrictions, be used, inspected, modified and redistributed [8]. Accelerates software development and adoption rates by enabling users to coordinate their efforts and leverage each other's contributions.

vii.   *User innovation*: Recognizes the fact that users are powerful innovators and often intuitively come up with good solutions to unidentified problems, both of which are easily overlooked from a vendor's point of view. Enables non-linear evolution of software and products. [9]

viii. *Distributed computing:* A field of computer science concerned with studying systems consisting of independent, networked computers and applications built across devices. Enhances resilience in computer systems through redundancy and loose coupling of computational nodes.

The proposed technological solution, which aims at realizing the key requirements (1-4) listed above by leveraging and implementing the above concepts (i-viii), is outlined next. Each device is equipped with a hypervisor, on top of which a common application platform is installed. The platform serves two main functions. First, it provides applications and services with a distributed deployment platform, which makes it possible to install the same piece of software on many different kinds of devices. This minimizes the need to maintain several different versions of a particular piece of software in order to support a wide variety of hardware. Second, the platform implements a management interface for maintaining the device, a set of APIs and supporting services, for example middleware services for discovering and interoperating with other devices and applications installed on them. Below is a list of example functionality that the platform might provide:

- *Device management interface:* Used for configuring and diagnosing the device and maintaining the list of known peers. For example, when initially setting up a device the interface can be used for configuring basic functionality such as networking services, device ids, and checking the list of auto-discovered peers and services.

- *Application management interface / Distributed community "app store":* Used for adding, removing and configuring installed applications. Applications are downloaded from other peers or dedicated application repositories. A key point here is that all applications that are installed on a device are automatically made available for other devices to download. This increases the resilience (see req. 4, above) of application availability and reduces the need for providing expensive bandwidth to popular applications, as the bandwidth burden is shared among all devices that have the particular application installed.
- *Inter-device communication*: A service that eases the application developer's burden of implementing peer device and/or application discovery and inter-communication facilities. This is especially important for distributed deployments of Web applications as they typically do not natively have this capability due to limitations inherent in the HTTP protocol and browser security restrictions (especially those meant for preventing cross-site scripting).
- *Privacy certificate verification:* Used for verifying the platform's authenticity (using its privacy certificate) and that it is installed on top of an untampered hypervisor or hardware. Also used for verifying the privacy certificates of all 3rd-party applications installed on the device.
- *Privacy toolkit:* Provides a pre-installed set of APIs and services aimed at application developers which ease implementation of privacy-preserving data storage, handling and dissemination functionality. For example by ensuring that dissemination of data is only performed using authorized and safe privacy policies or that all data is automatically equipped with expiration dates that are unconditionally enforced.

Additionally, an associated transparent, non-profit and ideally donations-funded organization run by the community and dedicated solely to the furthering of privacy-preserving ubiquitous computing would be needed. It might provide the following services to the public:

- Coordinating development efforts aimed at providing people with the aforementioned application platform and ensuring that it is compatible and easy to install on available commodity hardware.
- Providing a venue for enabling open code review of the platform and applications as well as requesting, issuing and revocation of privacy certificates.
- Educating the public regarding privacy issues and their implications in ubiquitous computing.
- Supporting community-driven ubiquitous computing application development and sharing.

4   Methodological Approach

The methodological approach of the author's thesis work is outlined, stage-by-stage, below. Six distinct stages are described but they are not meant to strictly follow each other, instead they are intended to be progressively refined in an iterative manner.

First, a conceptual framework of the community-driven ubiquitous computing ecology as proposed above is drawn out in detail. This includes the general architectural composition of the software appliance-based application platform and its basic services, application development, deployment and sharing schemes, privacy certification and verification process, role and functions of the ecology's coordinating entity and other associated parties, as well the relationships between them.

Second, an application domain within ubiquitous computing is selected for which a technological proof-of-concept implementation of the platform, and a few example applications are created with which the proposed solution's feasibility is to be initially evaluated and refined. The results from the particular testing domain should ideally be generalizable to the field of ubiquitous computing in general.

Third, the platform, along with the sample applications, is deployed in a live environment and initial tests with real test subjects are carried out. This is to verify the practical feasibility of the approach.

Fourth, 3rd party developers are invited to develop applications for the platform and deploy them in a live environment for ordinary users to try out. This is to test the feasibility of the community-driven application development approach.

Fifth, the application platform is released to the public for testing the feasibility of extending the hardware infrastructure using community efforts and commodity hardware. Emphasis should be placed on making the setup and maintenance of the infrastructure as straightforward as possible.

Sixth, final tests and surveys of the whole concept are carried out, including user and developer interviews and analyses of logs collected during the live tests. The rate of diffusion might also be considered as a potentially important indicator of the impact of the proposed approach.

5   UbiOulu Research

Stages one and two were to some degree already begun before the author's work in this field began. As the research has progressed, these have iteratively been refined, but the evaluation application domain of public displays has largely stayed the same. Public/ambient displays is a subfield of ubiquitous computing and is convenient in the sense that it resembles traditional computing to a large degree, while retaining UbiComp's special characteristic of having computation "fade into the background". The general concept and its approach, as outlined in this paper, should also be applicable to the field as a whole.

In stage three we deployed a large test bed network of public displays in downtown Oulu, Finland, equipped them with the application platform and some proof-of-concept Web-based distributed applications and exposed them to the public scrutiny of the citizens of Oulu. [10] In stage four, we invited members of the public to develop applications for our displays and published them among our own applications. Stage five is still work-in-progress, but is nearing completion, after which it will be released to the community for public scrutiny. Stage six is still at the planning stage.

6 Conclusion

In this paper a conceptual framework for enabling community-driven, extensible, open and privacy-preserving ubiquitous computing networks was presented. It leverages the results from several subfields including privacy-preserving computing, user innovation, free software, living labs, distributed computing as well as distributed web applications.

The author's thesis work is important to the field of ubiquitous computing, as it may set a precedent that will hopefully influence future research to take privacy issues and the power of the community into account to a larger degree in the future. It is the author's belief that privacy-preserving measures should be implemented as a pre-emptive measure, before ubiquitous computing becomes mainstream technology. Bolting-on privacy in hindsight may be difficult due to the large ubiquitous computing infrastructures and value networks that will at that point already have been set up.

References

1. Langheinrich, M.: Privacy in Ubiquitous Computing. In: Krumm, J. (ed.) Ubiquitous Computing Fundamentals, 1st edn. Chapman & Hall/CRC (2010)
2. Solove, D.J.: The Virtues of Knowing Less: Justifying Privacy Protections Against Disclosure. Duke Law Journal 53, 967 (2003)
3. Weiser, M.: The Computer for the 21st Century- Scientific American Special Issue on Communications, Computers, and Networks (September 1991)
4. Agrawal, R., Imieliński, T., Swami, A.: Mining association rules between sets of items in large databases. SIGMOD Rec. 22(2), 207–216 (1993), doi:10.1145/170036.170072
5. Taipale, K.A.: Data Mining and Domestic Security: Connecting the Dots to Make Sense of Data. Columbia Science and Technology Law Review 5(2) (December 2003)
6. Cranor, L.F., Reagle, J., Ackerman, M.S.: Beyond concern: Understanding net users' attitudes about online privacy. Technical Report TR 99.4.3, AT&T Labs-Research (April 1999)
7. Verykios, V.S., Bertino, E., Fovino, I.N., Provenza, L.P., Saygin, Y., Theodoridis, Y.: State-of-the-art in privacy preserving data mining. SIGMOD Rec. 33(1), 50–57 (2004)
8. Stallman, R.M.: Free Software, Free Society: Selected Essays of Richard M. Stallman, 2nd edn. GNU Press, Boston (2010); ISBN 978-0-9831592-0-9
9. von Hippel, E.: Democratizing Innovation. MIT Press (2005)
10. Ojala, T., Kukka, H., Lindén, T., Heikkinen, T., Jurmu, M., Hosio, S., Kruger, F.: UBI-Hotspot 1.0: Large-Scale Long-Term Deployment of Interactive Public Displays in a City Center. In: Fifth International Conference on Internet and Web Applications and Services (ICIW), pp. 285–294 (2010)

Doctoral Colloquium: Integrating Web Content into Mashups on Desktop and Mobile Devices

Arto Salminen

Department of Software Systems
Tampere University of Technology
P.O. Box 553, FIN-33101 Tampere, Finland
arto.salminen@tut.fi

Abstract. Mashups, web application hybrids that combine content from different services, are exploiting pervasiveness of the Internet and offering great value for the end user. Constantly evolving web technologies and new web services open up unforeseen possibilities for mashup development. Combining dynamic scripts with binary software is an interesting option. However, developing mashups with current methods and tools for existing deployment environments is challenging. This work concentrates on these challenges and finds ways to solve and circumvent issues related to mashups. Another important topic is analyzing the impact of new web technologies on mashup development. This research presents the mashups as a new breed of web applications that are intended for parsing the web content into easily accessed form on both regular computers as well as on other platforms, e.g. on embedded devices.

Keywords: mashups, web applications, web technologies, mobile devices.

1   Introduction

The Web has become pervasive. It is accessible from everywhere, available for everybody and used for everything. This has led to a paradigm shift, where applications live on the Web as services. Moreover, different kinds of devices can be used to get access to these services, including – in addition to regular computers – many kinds of embedded devices, such as mobile phones, game consoles, and so forth. We believe that this is only the beginning of a new era, where the Web is a ubiquitous distribution channel for data, code and other content.

Applications built on top of the web do not have to live by the same constraints that conventional desktop software. The ability to dynamically combine content from numerous web sites and local resources, and the ability to instantly publish services worldwide has opened up entirely new possibilities for software development. In general, such systems are referred to as mashups, which are content aggregates that leverage the power of the Web to support instant, worldwide sharing of content.

Traditional mashups are executed inside a web browser but other systems can be used as a runtime environment as well. A mashup can combine the content in new,

M. Rautiainen et al. (Eds.): GPC 2011 Workshops, LNCS 7096, pp. 164–171, 2012.

unforeseen way, thus creating entirely new web service, or a mashup can provide new visualization for existing service. Typically mashups are divided into two categories, client-side and server-side mashups, based on where downloading, processing and generating of the web content takes place.

However, there are numerous stumbling stones on the road of mashup developer. For instance, lack of well-defined interfaces and inadequate security model of browser-based applications makes mashup composing problematic. In addition, our experience has shown that mobile mashups struggle with usability, connectivity and performance problems.

Web browser is not the only execution environment for mashups. Especially when the target device is not regular computer, it might be practical to use custom runtime environments. Many mobile phone manufacturers have their own web application frameworks: Nokia's WRT Widgets and Apple's Web Apps, for instance. Furthermore, it is possible to create mashups by combining dynamic code and native binary libraries. This kind of hybrid approach has the flexibility of dynamic code and the performance of binary applications. However, it is still important to make research about what is the best way to divide functionality between static and dynamic parts of the application, and about how technical issues related to combinations of scripts and binaries can be solved.

New web technologies are offering great building blocks for composing web applications. For example, WebGL [4] is enabling 3D graphics API to be used inside a web browser without plugins, and HTML5 [5] is bringing support for embedded audio and video, cross-document messaging, offline storage database and local SQL database, among others. These are remarkable improvements that will gear the web browser into more and more powerful platform for complex applications. From mashup development point of view these tools can enable compositions that are yet completely unforeseen.

This paper is structured as follows. Section 2 provides an overview of related work in the area of the PhD work. Then, in section 3, we present the research objectives and specific problems addressed and describe the methodology used to pursue the objectives. In section 4, we describe the research already carried out and the contributions made in the field of pervasive computing. Finally, in section 5, we summarize this paper.

2   Related Work

Numerous mashup applications have already been developed and deployed. Handful of tools, intended for mashup composition, has been introduced. Current mashup research has been focusing on mashup applications and browser-based frameworks. Some work has already been done on the field of mashup security. On the following we will briefly describe the related work.

2.1   Mashup Application Examples

A simple example of a communication mashup is Nokia N900 device's instant messaging application. It can be used to make connections to several communication services such as Facebook chat, SIP account, Microsoft Messenger, Google Talk or Skype. The application has support for add-ons so it can be easily expanded to handle new services.

Google has created a mashup called Google Maps for Mobile (*http://www. google.com/mobile/maps/*), whose main component is a map that shows the user's current GPS location. This mashup system can be used to track positions of friends and to display additional map related information, including traffic data, driving directions, interesting places or web camera images, on layers over the map.

Another interesting example of mobile map-based mashup is Telar Mashup for Nokia N810 tablet by Brodt et al. [6]. It uses modified mobile web browser to gain an access to GPS peripheral of the device and combines the location data with map retrieved from Google Maps.

2.2   Mashup Tools

Tobias Nestler has done research [7] about Service Oriented Architectures from the Service-to-User point of view. He pointed out that existing mashup tools such as Yahoo (*http://pipes.yahoo.com/pipes/*), Microsoft Popfly (discontinued during autumn 2009) and IBM QedWiki (*http://www01.ibm.com/software/info/mashup-center/*) are lacking support for input and output parameters other than simple data types. Another discovery was that UI components such as buttons, navigation elements or multiple screens, were not supported in existing tools.

Technical report by Antero Taivalsaari [8] lists a number of existing mashup development tools which are geared towards ordinary users instead of just professional programmers. Most of the tools described support programming via some kind of visual programming interface but allow source code editing as an advanced feature.

Research [9] by Wang et al. describes end-user mashup programming using nested tables and designing a developing environment that uses this approach. The programming model of the environment relies on spreadsheet-style view for the mashup data. The data inside worksheets can be modified with simple scripts that consist of very limited set of operations.

Cao et al. studied end-user mashup designing [10] by conducting a think-aloud experiment with ten participants creating a web mashup using the Microsoft Popfly mashup tool already mentioned above. They discovered that participants designed their mashups by numerous iterations divided into framing, acting and reflecting phases. Another discovery was that presenting application logic alongside with the runtime output and providing visual hints about connection between those two would have made the debugging task a lot easier.

2.3   Mashup Frameworks

De et al. have developed a mashup framework called Service Context Manager (SCM) framework [11]. SCM handles all the stages of context gathering, processing, inferring and reasoning to come up with useful recommendations. It consists of three parts: 1) device and service discovery function, 2) transformation framework and 3) reasoning module.

Ikeda et al. [12] have designed a framework for creating flexible mashups in which the user can selectively browse through mashup items. The framework includes data management engine for on-demand data generation and GUI widgets that can be used to browse the data. These are both implemented on client-side as well as connections to different web services. On the server-side the framework provides only configuration files for widgets and data management.

2.4   Mashup Security

Service access control API that aims to better mashup security has been studied by Hashimoto et al. [13]. The SAXAE API provides functions to the mashup to retrieve protected, non-public resources securely This allows the mashup to access user's private data, for example on some social service, in secure fashion.

Warner et al. have researched privacy protection model for government mashups [14]. This model allows users to specify their individual privacy policies that can be applied to the use of their data. The approach involves the protection of sensitive data based on not only who is requesting access but on the intended use too.

Another security related studies are lattice-based mashup security model by Magazinius et al. [15]. The security lattice is build from the origins of mashup components so that the each level of the lattice corresponds to a set of origins. To allow a controlled release of information between mashup components, a declassification mechanism is proposed. Declassification policy defines what pieces of information can be shared between components. Sharing data from security level to another can only be done if it is allowed explicitly.

An identity management protocol for mashups has been studied by Zarandioon et al. [16]. Their proposal utilizes conventional public-key cryptography to eliminate need for a trusted identify provider. In addition, their research describes a framework that allows secure indirect communication between client-side mashup components. Both the identity management protocol and the framework are implemented as an in-browser library.

3   Research Objectives and Methodology

The research problems to be examined are related to issues around mashups, changes on the field of mashup development, different platforms where mashups are useful and designing mashups in combination with binary software. After defining the research questions, we describe the research methodology.

3.1   Research Questions

Background study clearly shows that the mashups can be constructed in numerous different ways with a plethora of tools, and there still are major practical problems related to mashup composing and security. For instance, the web browser security model is too restricting for mashups, tools introduced are lacking behind, and using dynamic languages for large applications is unknown territory for many developers. The field of web programming is constantly changing as new interfaces, technologies and frameworks build upon novel technologies emerge constantly. The amount of different, constantly evolving APIs with different licenses is overwhelming. When developing large-scale mashups, situation may be even more problematic. Therefore, some general guidelines may be found to be able to handle this diversified situation. Furthermore, numerous other runtime environments than a web browser that may benefit mashup development have been introduced. This leads to the first research question (RQ1):

RQ1. How to solve or facilitate problems related to mashup development?

While mobility sets restrictions to applications and application development, at the same time it is a great opportunity from mashup development point of view. The dynamic nature of mashups suits well for different ways mobile terminals can be used. Often, the information needed on the fly is related to user's context, which can be available for applications to access automatically [3]. This opens up opportunities to provide advantageous user experiences, as mashups can dynamically present eligible information, possibly even automatically without requiring specific user action. However, as mobile devices capabilities are limited, extending mashups to mobile domain is not trivial. Special solutions, such as runtime environments and support from powerful server architecture for mobile clients, may be needed. This derives to the second question (RQ2):

RQ2. What opportunities and restrictions are associated with mashups in mobile devices?

There are situations when composition of a mashup is not possible using only dynamic code. For example, applications, that require a lot of computation power or access to interfaces that are not available for dynamic code, have to be constructed with both dynamic and native code. Therefore, offering an interface for mixing web technologies with the capabilities of native software components can be used as a platform for composing complex applications that combine the best of both worlds: performance and eye candy of traditional, installed binary applications and pervasiveness and seemingly infinite resources of the web. Implementation of this kind of hybrid mashups leads to the third question (RQ3):

RQ3. How mashups benefit when native binary software is combined with dynamic code both on desktop and on embedded devices?

As results, we expect to have broader and deeper view into mashups in general, broad understanding about current situation of mashup problems, practical solutions to issues that developers face when designing mashups, guidelines to follow when designing mashups, couple of environments for mashup development (both embedded systems and desktop computers), and practical approach to combine scripts and binary software.

3.2   Research Methodology

Constructive research methods have been applied in developing the mashups and mashup infrastructure and empirical methods in the application evaluation. In addition, case studies may be used in the artifact evaluation. With constructive methods, we examine mashups on numerous platforms, both on desktop and on embedded devices. Furthermore, we examine systems build with hybrid approach referred in RQ3.

4   Research Carried Out and Contributions

As a part of a larger activity called *Lively for Qt* (*http://lively.cs.tut.fi/qt*) – a project that has created a highly interactive, mobile web application and mashup development environment for the Qt cross-platform application framework – we developed a variety of mashups. Using the Lively for Qt platform instead of a web browser allows creating the applications without restrictions of the web browser. Even though a special runtime is used, result mashups can be run in a web browser if a plug-in component is installed. As a result we found out a number of issues related to mashups in the areas of usability, connectivity and performance. The platform used, was found successful as a mobile mashup platform. These results are described in [2].

Another early research effort, documented in [1], was creating mashups that run inside the web browser as well as inside the Lively for Qt environment. Based on our experiences we provided a set of guidelines and "recipes" for successful mashup development. These guidelines were about mashup design, interfacing with web services as well as some broader issues.

Using a Qt-based runtime environment, we created a mashup platform [3] – written in pure JavaScript – that had access to device peripherals using standardized interfaces available in the device. Using the platform, we created a simple example application that could access a mobile device's GPS peripherals and share the user location and status messages collaboratively with other users. The platform enables mashups that have liberal and flexible access to device resources as well as infinite resources of the web to be realized.

The idea of platform allowing context aware mashups was later expanded, as we created mashups using a hybrid technique where applications had both binary and dynamic parts [17]. While previous mashups were developed with procedural application development style, now a declarative approach was used. This hybrid approach enabled high performance client side mashups, which could have access to device peripherals in even more liberate fashion compared to the previous pure JavaScript solution [3].

It is obvious that when large scale mashups with tens of thousands of content items and users are developed, new challenges will emerge. Therefore, we designed a mashup ecosystem [18], which was later realized as mashup architecture [19]. Evaluation of the architecture is still under way, but a video mashup client developed for Android platform as the first prototype using this architecture seems promising.

Currently the thesis work has emphasis on writing the dissertation introduction and composing a focused and clear presentation about the research results. A journal paper that deepens ideas presented in [1] is currently under way. However, the research work around the topic continues with exploring the novel web technologies, such as HTML5 and WebGL. It seems that HTML5 as well as WebGL have a great impact on mashup development and on the web programming in general. With WebGL, 3D and other visually rich mashups can be composed without web browser's cumbersome DOM interface and with much better performance. Furthermore, the HTML5 enables a variety of things that we are used to on desktop applications, such as drag-and-drop, local databases, file access, video, sound and web workers (threads), that will be very useful on mashup development.

Our future efforts around mashups include creating a 3D mashup environment, developing an environment for so called ambient mashups and composing a mashup architecture, which allows different vendors to contribute in a "living" mashup ecosystem. The 3D mashup environment is build with HTML5 and WebGL and it can contain both 2D and 3D web applications. The environment contains programming tools that can be used to create new applications or combine and expand existing applications. Ambient mashups are automatically acquiring information about the user surroundings using device sensors and other peripherals. This way mashup content can be updated without user interaction. Mashup architecture is a large scale description of the operational environment of different actors producing web services and others creating mashups that use these services. Having a well-structured architecture is important when the target is to compose mashups that are efficient as well as maintainable and used for real tasks in contrast to being just opportunistic hacks.

5   Summary

It is clear that combining content from multiple sources can utilize the pervasiveness of the web in a powerful fashion. However, research already done in this field -- by us and other researchers -- clearly shows that numerous problems are still unsolved. We believe that as technical problems are solved, mashups will be a very practical tool for personal and enterprise use, when relevant information needs to be expressed in simple, effective and illustrative way.

References

1. Salminen, A., Nyrhinen, F., Mikkonen, T., Taivalsaari, A.: Developing Client-Side Mashups: Experiences, Guidelines and the Road Ahead. In: Proc. of the MindTrek 2010 Conference (MindTrek 2010), Tampere, Finland (2010)
2. Nyrhinen, F., Salminen, A., Mikkonen, T., Taivalsaari, A.: Lively mashups for mobile devices. In: Proc. of the First Int. Conf. on Mobile Computing, Applications and Services, San Diego, CA (2009)
3. Mikkonen, T., Salminen, A.: Towards pervasive mashups in embedded devices. In: Proceedings of the 16th IEEE International Conference on Embedded and Real-Time Computing Systems and Applications, pp. 35–42. IEEE Computer Society (2010)

4. Khronos Group. WebGL Specification. technical specification (February 10, 2011), `http://www.khronos.org/registry/webgl/specs/1.0/` (retrieved March 17, 2011)
5. World Wide Web Consortium. A vocabulary and associated APIs for HTML and XHTML. technical specification (January 13, 2011), `http://www.w3.org/TR/html5/` (retrieved March 17, 2011)
6. Brodt, A., Nicklas, D.: The TELAR mobile mashup platform for Nokia internet tablets. In: Proceedings of 11th International Conference on Extending Database Technology, Munich, Germany (2008)
7. Nestler, T.: Towards a mashup-driven end-user programming of SOA-based applications. In: Proceedings of the 10th International Conference on Information Integration and Web-Based Applications & Services, Linz, Austria, November 24-26 (2008)
8. Wang, G., Yang, S., Han, Y.: Mashroom: end-user mashup programming using nested tables. In: Proceedings of the 18th International Conference on World Wide Web, Madrid, Spain (2009)
9. Taivalsaari, A.: Mashware: The Future of Web Applications. Sun Microsystems Laboratories, Technical Report TR-2009-181 (2009)
10. Cao, J., Riche, Y., Wiedenbeck, S., Burnett, M., Grigoreanu, V.: End-user mashup programming: through the design lens. In: Proceedings of the 28th International Conference on Human Factors in Computing Systems, Atlanta, Georgia, USA (2010)
11. De, S., Moessner, K.: A framework for mobile, context-aware applications. In: Proceedings of the 16th International Conference on Telecommunications, Marrakech, Morocco (2009)
12. Ikeda, S., Nagamine, T., Kamada, T.: Application framework with demand-driven mashup for selective browsing. In: Proceedings of the 10th International Conference on Information Integration and Web-Based Applications & Services, Linz, Austria (2008)
13. Hashimoto, R., Ueno, N., Shimomura, M.: A design of usable and secure access-control APIs for mashup applications. In: Proceedings of the 5th ACM Workshop on Digital Identity Management, Chicago, Illinois, USA, November 13 (2009)
14. Warner, J., Chun, S.A.: A citizen privacy protection model for e-government mashup services. In: Proceedings of the 2008 International Conference on Digital Government Research, Montreal, Canada (2008)
15. Magazinius, J., Askarov, A., Sabelfeld, A.: A lattice-based approach to mashup security. In: Proceedings of the 5th ACM Symposium on information, Computer and Communications Security, Beijing, China (2010)
16. Zarandioon, S., Yao, D., Ganapathy, V.: Privacy-aware identity management for client-side mashup applications. In: Proceedings of the 5th ACM Workshop on Digital Identity Management, Chicago, Illinois, USA (2009)
17. Salminen, A., Mikkonen, T.: Towards Pervasive Mashups in Embedded Devices: Comparing Procedural and Declarative Approach. Under review
18. Salminen, A., Kallio, J., Mikkonen, T.: Towards Mobile Multimedia Mashup Ecosystem. To appear in Proceedings of IEEE ICC 2011 Workshop on Advances in Mobile Networking - Towards a Next Generation Mobile Core Network, ICC 2011, Kyoto, Japan (2011)
19. Hartikainen, M., Salminen, A., Kallio, J., Mikkonen, T.: Towards Mashup Ecosystem Architecture. In: Under review for SEAA 2011 Conference in Oulu, Finland (2011)

Lightweight Service-Based Software Architecture

Mikko Polojärvi and Jukka Riekki

Intelligent Systems Group and Infotech Oulu
University of Oulu, Oulu, Finland
{mikko.polojarvi,jukka.riekki}@ee.oulu.fi

Abstract. This article describes the Simple Event Relaying Framework (SERF), a novel service-based software architecture designed especially for resource constrained settings and facilitated cooperation between applications. The proposed prototype framework aims at utilizing publish/ subscribe and peer-to-peer, technologies that are usually encountered only in higher level inter-device networks, inside the software architecture of individual applications in very simple form. The idea is to introduce a simple core architecture on which more advanced features can be built on. The research will be conducted primarily by creating prototype solutions to real life problems and learning from the experience.

1 Introduction

One trend in information technology nowadays is that modern mobile devices are more and more composed of larger number of small applications. One smart phone might easily contain over one hundred user-installed applications. We can consider the applications networked to some degree, but often they are still quite separated from each other. They seldom communicate or cooperate with each other, and even if they do, it is usually done only in the way the application developers have specifically envisioned.

This does not need to be limited to the software inside a single mobile device. For example, in Smart Space research everyday environment is envisioned as full of networked smart objects, or miniature computers or sensors that fulfill a very specific purpose, for example detecting the user's presence in a room. This information alone is not useful alone, it needs to be combined with an application that can use the information in some way, for example by turning the lights on. In the same way as above, it is neither possible for the smart object designers to know all the ways the information could be utilized, nor possible for the application designers to know all the future devices that could provide the information. This is a problem that limits the usefulness of the smart space applications and objects.

We could argue same applies to individual applications as well. Applications usually consist of a number of smaller software components, and if we consider memory references, function calls etc. as links, we can consider the software components networked. While running, these components do lot of information

M. Rautiainen et al. (Eds.): GPC 2011 Workshops, LNCS 7096, pp. 172–179, 2012.

processing. If the application developer cannot think of a reason to expose the results of this processing outside, the results probably will not be available to other applications, since building for such flexibility usually also consumes resources.

Therein lies great potential for development. If software components could be made to open up more efficiently for cooperation with each other, it would open the way for using applications in many ways not originally planned for. In order to allow such unplanned cooperation between applications, the internal state of the applications needs to be implicitly exposed outside the application.

One solution could be to make even the smallest component loosely coupled and communicate using the publish/subscribe paradigm. Each component would have clear cut purpose in the application and depend very little or not at all on other components in order to fulfill the purpose. The components would send (i.e. publish) messages around so that only the components that have expressed interest (i.e. subscribed) in a certain message type end up receiving them. Senders would not care who they are sending to, and receivers would not care where they get the messages from, as long as the content of the message is interesting. As a result, senders and receivers could be freely added, removed, moved or modified without breaking the whole system, allowing the components to cooperate with each other in unforeseeable ways.

Naturally, within the idea there are many challenges, but first and foremost is the question of how to organize the communication between the components in practice? The QoS requirements for communication at different levels (inside an application, between applications, between devices etc.) vary greatly. There already exist numerous solutions utilizing publish/subscribe, but most existing solutions are aimed at large scale inter-device networks and often assume a single mobile device as the smallest unit in the network of components. Many publish/subscribe solutions are simply too heavy computationally for use in lower level communications, services and algorithms. This is further aggravated by the fact that in mobile devices, power, storage and computing resources are considerably limited. Other challenges are discussed later.

This is where my doctoral thesis research comes in. The research investigates the possibility of utilizing publish/subscribe in considerably lower level settings, with the aim of allowing unplanned cooperation between components. Towards this purpose I have developed a novel component based general purpose software framework prototype called the Simple Event Relaying Framework (SERF). SERF is a continuation of my earlier work, the Ideasilo framework published in [1]. This particular prototype concentrates in the software architecture inside individual applications. In this paper I will explain the detailed design, experiences received thus far, research methods and expected results of my work. But first, I will present a review about other related solutions.

2   Related Work

Service Oriented Architecture (SOA) is one prominent modern tool utilizing loosely coupled modules. In fact, the current SERF prototype has been largely inspired by the principles of SOA [6]. Most of the principles have been adopted unchanged or in slightly modified form. However, some principles have been discarded in order to accommodate usage in resource constrained settings.

Android's Intent system [3] is also meant to facilitate inter-component cooperation within a single mobile device. An intent is a passive data structure holding an abstract definition of an operation to be performed or a description of something that has happened. In case a component interested in the service is not loaded by the time the intent is executed, the system automatically instantiates them.

Among experimental solutions, Network on Terminal Architecture (NoTA) [4], developed in the Nokia Research Center and first released in 2005, bears some similarities with SERF. Both are have a similar purpose (facilitate software development) and solution principle (use SOA in device level settings). The Smart-M3 [5] project is similar in the sense that it also aims at software cooperation at multiple levels, but concerns itself mostly on inter-device part. Both NoTA and Smart-M3 differ greatly from SERF in design, and neither use publish/subscribe in messaging by itself.

3   Proposed Solution

As stated before, SERF is designed for investigating the possibility of utilizing publish/subscribe also within low level software components. The current prototype concentrates primarily in resource-wise the most demanding part, communication between components inside individual applications, while keeping a secondary focus on inter-application and inter-device communication. Therefore the design concentrates in providing the communication framework with as few resources as possible.

SERF addresses the challenges of designing general purpose software frameworks by making very few assumptions about the used technologies or applications built upon it, and not trying to do too much. In fact, in my approach SERF aims at providing just a conceptual answer the question: "which message should be delivered to which components?"

The SERF research is based on the following hypotheses:

1. Working and useful applications can be formed using primarily loosely coupled components with less resources than creating every component from scratch.
2. Higher level framework functionality can be implemented as applications on top of a very simple core framework.
3. It is possible for different applications to cooperate in new ways that have not been taken into account at design time.
4. Lightweight messaging architecture can offer significant reductions in computational workload as compared to more feature-rich solutions.

The design of the first prototype of SERF is described in detail at [2]. Although the current solution features an upgraded scheduling solution, most of the design principles and implementation still apply to the current prototype. A brief summary of the design is presented next. The main principles of the current approach can be summarized as follows:

1. The framework is kept as simple as possible.
2. The main idea of the framework is conceptual and platform-independent.
3. An application is composed of a many small components that send messages to each other.
4. The components form an acyclic network with each other.
5. The framework will route messages from the sender to the recipient(s) by the topic of the message. The framework will not concern itself with the identity of the sender of the recipient.
6. Messages will not describe what should happen in the application. Instead, the messages simply describe what is happening at the moment. Other components may then decide how to act on the information.
7. The framework concentrates on keeping the overhead of routing the messages from senders to receivers at minimum.

Figure 1 presents an example about the current component structure. The structure consists of event processors, routers and filters, and thread schedulers. Event processors ($P_1 - P_5$ in the figure) can be understood as the application components mentioned earlier. These are developed by the application designers using the framework. Real applications are formed by having them communicate with each other. They are basically pieces of code that generate and receive messages, the framework being responsible for executing the event handling code when necessary.

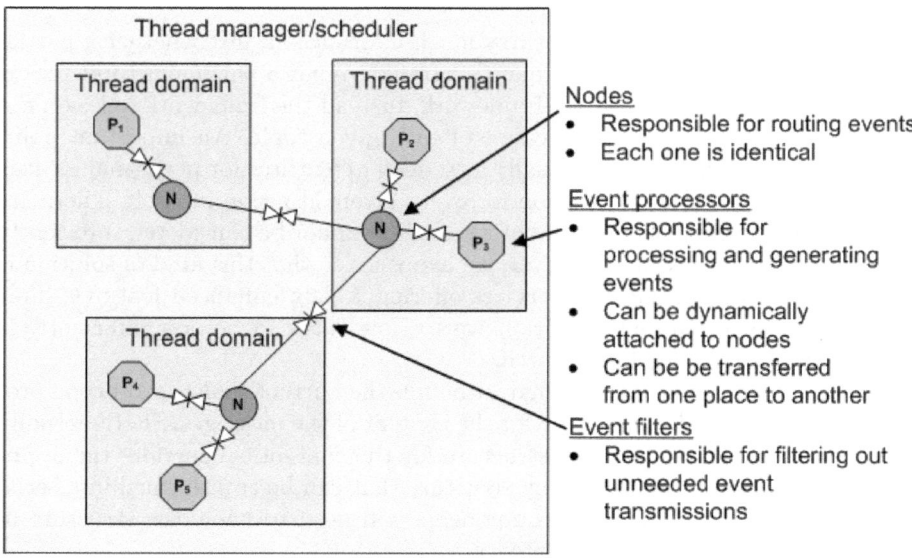

Fig. 1. SERF routing example

Routing nodes (the N:s) in figure 1 are responsible for routing the messages to processors and other routing nodes. These are all identical to each other, although their configuration may differ. When necessary, the thread scheduler (the surrounding big box) assigns a thread to work at each node demanding attention. The thread routes messages, executes processors and returns to wait for more work on other nodes. The solution ensures that all processors attached to the same node are always executed in the same thread (as indicated by the Thread Domain box around each node). One important aspect of this solution is that this kind of structure supports multi-processor architecture in the sense that it encourages dividing the application into clear cut components. Each component can be easily assigned to be worked on by a separate processor core, and the number of worker threads can be easily adjusted. The event-based messaging design also inherently reduces many concurrency problems usually associated with thread-based programming.

The event filters (the diode signs) in figure 1 are responsible for handling the actual routing of messages. Each link from router to router or router to processor contains two filters, one for each direction. Every message contains meta information about the topic of the message, where a single topic is represented with a single bit in a particular position in an array of bytes. This way the demands of a complete branch of nodes in the network can be represented in compact form with byte arrays and evaluated efficiently with binary operators. These filter evaluations are repeated once for each link in a routing node. Because in SERF the routing node network cannot contain loops, this potentially results in larger logical distance between the nodes as compared to cyclic networks. However, if the overhead of a single filter check and event transmission can be kept sufficiently low, the overhead may still be less than by using more complex routing solutions.

Obviously a single bit cannot carry much information, just whether a particular topic applies to the event in question or not. What a particular topic means is not modeled in any way in the framework. Instead the framework relies on the designers agreeing on the significance of each given topic. An important point here is that this solution is essentially a tradeoff of features for performance. It is not intended to be perfect solution for every given situation in itself. There are indeed many cases where this kind of messaging cannot be considered sufficiently scalable, robust or flexible. However, we hypothesize that this kind of solution is still able to support a layer of services offering widely enhanced features, built on top of the very simple core framework. How this can be done efficiently is another promising topic for research.

An important notion here is that although the current SERF prototype provides a simple key-value structure for the content of the messages, SERF actually does not assume any particular structure for the contents. Therefore the application designers are free to use any structure that can be transformed into serial form, although communicating components will need to know the structure in order to be able to access the contents.

4   Methods

In the next phase of my research I intend to evaluate the possibility of utilizing publish/subscribe in low level settings by searching answers to the following research questions:

1. What kind of advantages can be achieved by applying lightweight publish/subscribe in low-level settings?
2. What disadvantages does the above have? In order to achieve the benefits, what compromises must be made?
3. On what kind of application areas will the advantages outweigh the disadvantages?

In order to provide the answers, my approach is primarily based on experimenting with prototypes with the aim of gaining broadened understanding on using SERF in practice. The plan is to iterate the following workflow:

1. Based on literature review on the theory of software frameworks and messaging, and the experiences gained from the previous steps, develop and optimize the SERF framework.
2. Discover a real life problem where the current SERF framework could be utilized to a desirable effect. Here the choice of the problem area does not need to be limited only to resource constrained settings, as it is valuable to study how well SERF performs also in less resource constrained settings.
3. Study the theory related to the problem area at hand and different kinds of possible solutions.
4. Develop a prototype solution to the aforementioned real life problem using SERF and software components required by the application, preferably ones already created earlier in the workflow. Also, when possible, a second solution using another feasible competing solution should be implemented for comparison.
5. Evaluate the prototype quantitatively by benchmarking and qualitatively by user tests, compare the results to competing solutions and publish the findings.

This plan provides good opportunities for interdisciplinary research collaboration. Moreover, the workflow itself serves as a sanity check on the main hypotheses presented earlier. The workflow also works as an experiment on how easily software components made earlier in the workflow can be utilized in later projects without essentially modifying the components and without knowing what a given component is going to be used for later.

As SERF is still in prototype stage, there are still many possibilities for further improvement. A fundamental question here is deciding which improvements should be implemented in the framework itself and which in the application layer, and which improvements rejected outright. Among others, the following possibilities will need consideration:

1. Similar to Android, the framework could support instantiation of event routers and processors when needed.
2. The framework could support mobile software components, i.e. pieces of code that are sent to remote devices for execution.
3. The event filtering solution could be still improved. Especially, utilizing Bloom filters [7] instead of byte arrays in the filtering solution could offer performance advantages.

5   Expected Results

There are many challenges associated with intra device software ecosystems, some of which I do not expect to be discovered without experimentation. For example, it can be expected that some information must not leak outside known application boundaries. Considering the idea of the framework is to share information implicitly, how should this be solved? Another challenge is to find a way to ensure that even with groving number of applications, the routing solution scales and individual applications do not conflict with each other. Managing multiple software components answering the same service request may also present a problem.

Although a working software framework prototype has already been developed, my research is still on relatively early stages, so the final course for the research is not yet completely fixed. The work presented in this paper can be understood as the first phase that will provide understanding on the challenges associated with using SERF for intra-application communication. In the current plan, the second phase will concentrate on studying the inter-application part.

In short, the ultimate aim of the research is to gain heightened understanding on the challenges associated with unplanned cooperation among software components. Secondarily, the aim is to provide a feasible and working software framework prototype for further work on the topic. Third, the described workflow will provide a number of smaller prototype applications, each providing insight into the application area in question.

6   Conclusion

In this article I have presented my doctoral thesis topic: SERF, a simple service-based software framework utilizing publish/subscribe in low level settings. The purpose of the framework is to facilitate cooperation between individual applications and software components. I have presented my reasoning why a simpler messaging framework is needed. I have described the current framework prototype and explained the reasons for main design principles. I have explained my plan for continuing the work on developing and evaluating the framework. Finally, I have described my expectations for the result of my research.

References

1. Polojärvi, M.: Application framework for utilizing RFID information Master's thesis, University of Oulu, Oulu, Finland (2008) (in Finnish)
2. Polojärvi, M., Riekki, J.: Experiences in Lightweight Event Relaying Framework Design Proceedings of FutureTech-10, Busan, Korea (2010)
3. Android, Developer Guide: Intents and Intent Filters, http://developer.android.com/guide/topics/intents/intents-filters.html
4. Nokia Research Center, NoTA Architecture, http://www.notaworld.org/nota/architecture
5. SourceForge, Smart-M3, http://sourceforge.net/projects/smart-m3/
6. Thomas Erl, The Service-Orientation Design Paradigm, http://www.soaprinciples.com/p3.php
7. Broder, A., Mitzenmacher, M.: Network Application of Bloom Filters: A Survey Internet Mathematics, vol. 1(4), pp. 485–509

Author Index